CLINICAL PROBLEM SOLVING IN
ORTHODONTICS
AND PAEDIATRIC
DENTISTRY

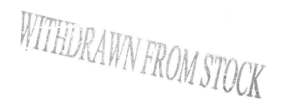

WITHDRAWN FROM STOCK

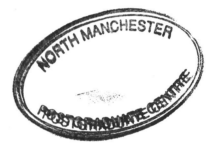

NORTH MANCHESTER
POSTGRADUATE CENTRE

D1394065

Commissioning Editor: Michael Parkinson
Project Development Manager: Lynn Watt
Project Manager: Frances Affleck
Designer: Erik Bigland
Illustration Manager: Bruce Hogarth

CLINICAL PROBLEM SOLVING IN
ORTHODONTICS AND PAEDIATRIC DENTISTRY

Declan Millett BDSc DDS FDSRCPS (Glasg) DOrthRCSEng MOrthRCSEng

Professor of Orthodontics
University College Cork
Ireland

Richard Welbury MB BS BDS PhD FDSRCS FDSRCPS FRCPCH

Professor of Paediatric Dentistry
University of Glasgow
UK

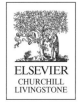

ELSEVIER
CHURCHILL
LIVINGSTONE

EDINBURGH   LONDON   NEW YORK   OXFORD   PHILADELPHIA   ST LOUIS   SYDNEY   TORONTO 2005

ELSEVIER
CHURCHILL
LIVINGSTONE

© 2005, Elsevier Limited. All rights reserved.

The right of Declan Millett and Richard Welbury to be identified as authors of this work has been asserted by them in accordance with the Copyright, Designs and Patents Act 1988.

No part of this publication may be reproduced, stored in a retrieval system, or transmitted in any form or by any means, electronic, mechanical, photocopying, recording or otherwise, without either the prior permission of the publishers or a licence permitting restricted copying in the United Kingdom issued by the Copyright Licensing Agency, 90 Tottenham Court Road, London W1T 4LP. Permissions may be sought directly from Elsevier's Health Sciences Rights Department in Philadelphia, USA: phone: (+1) 215 239 3804, fax: (+1) 215 239 3805, e-mail: healthpermissions@elsevier.com. You may also complete your request on-line via the Elsevier homepage (http://www.elsevier.com), by selecting 'Customer Support' and then 'Obtaining Permissions'.

First published 2005
  Reprinted 2005

ISBN 0 443 07265 5

British Library Cataloguing in Publication Data
A catalogue record for this book is available from the British Library

Library of Congress Cataloguing in Publication Data
A catalogue record for this book is available from the Library of Congress

Notice
Medical knowledge is constantly changing. Standard safety precautions must be followed, but as new research and clinical experience broaden our knowledge, changes in treatment and drug therapy may become necessary or appropriate. Readers are advised to check the most current product information provided by the manufacturer of each drug to be administered to verify the recommended dose, the method and duration of administration, and contraindications. It is the responsibility of the practitioner, relying on experience and knowledge of the patient, to determine dosages and the best treatment for each individual patient. Neither the Publisher nor the author assumes any liability for any injury and/or damage to persons or property arising from this publication.

The Publisher

ELSEVIER   your source for books,
journals and multimedia
in the health sciences
www.elsevierhealth.com

Working together to grow
libraries in developing countries
www.elsevier.com | www.bookaid.org | www.sabre.org

ELSEVIER   BOOKAID   Sabre Foundation
            International

The
publisher's
policy is to use
**paper manufactured
from sustainable forests**

Printed in China

Preface

Problem solving is a core skill which the dental undergraduate must develop and refine for examinations and everyday clinical practice. As orthodontics and paediatric dentistry interface broadly, combined clinical teaching and examinations in these disciplines are linked increasingly to encourage holistic problem solving of dental and occlusal problems in the child and adolescent patient.

This book aims, therefore, to address a range of common clinical problems encountered in orthodontic and paediatric dental practice. The format promotes a logical approach to problem solving through history taking, clinical examination and diagnosis, which underpain the principles of treatment planning for both disciplines. A short reference list is provided with each chapter to facilitate further directed learning.

Mind maps® are also given for each topic to provide a focused framework for learning and revision. Each mind map links key words, or key points, which are highlighted throughout the text, to create an overview of the subject and is designed to trigger information recall.

Intended primarily for the undergraduate, we hope this book will be of value also to the junior postgraduate and to those preparing for membership examinations.

DTM
RRW
Cork and Glasgow
2004

Acknowledgements

We are particularly grateful to Mrs K. Shepherd and Mrs G. Drake for their help and support in the preparation of photographic material. We would also like to thank especially Dr G. McIntyre, Ms R. Bryan, Mr J. C. Aird, Dr A. Shaw, Miss D. Fung and Mr S. A. Fayle for provision of some of the illustrations. Mr J. Brown also kindly assisted with the drawings of appliances. We are also grateful to Buzan Centres Ltd for the style for the Mind Maps.® Our gratitude is extended to the staff of Elsevier who have been very helpful throughout. We also thank Mrs A. Burson for drafting the the Mind Maps and Mrs R. Buttimer for her help with the bibliography. Finally, special tribute is due to Eithne Johnstone for her resolute and considerable skills, which greatly facilitated manuscript preparation.

Contents

1
Median diastema

Summary

Brian is almost 8 years of age. He presents with a gap between his upper front teeth and crooked lower front teeth (**Fig. 1.1**). What are the causes of these problems and what treatment would you recommend?

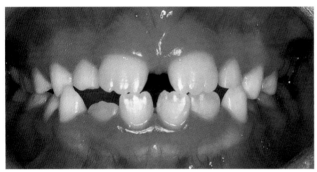

Fig. 1.1 Anterior occlusion at presentation.

History
● Complaint

Brian's mother noticed the gap between his upper front teeth and the irregularity of his lower front teeth. She is anxious about his appearance and is keen for treatment to be provided.

● History of complaint

Brian's primary front teeth had a pleasing appearance with a small midline space in the upper arch; the lower primary front teeth were not spaced. There is no history of trauma. The permanent incisors erupted in their present positions.

● Medical history

Brian is fit and well.

● Dental history

Brian attends his general dental practitioner every 6 months but has not required any treatment.

● Family history

Brian's father had an upper midline space that was closed with a fixed appliance.

Examination
● Extraoral examination

Brian has a Class I skeletal pattern with average FMPA and no facial asymmetry. Lips are competent with the lower lip resting at the incisal third of the upper central incisors. There are no temporomandibular joint signs or symptoms.

● Intraoral examination

Soft tissues are healthy and the dentition is caries-free. The intraoral views are shown in **Figures 1.1** and **1.2**.

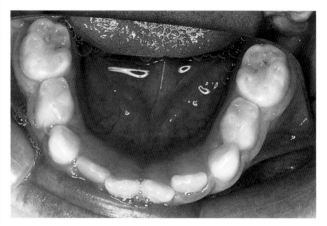

Fig. 1.2 Lower occlusal view (note $\overline{6|6}$ erupted but not shown).

What do you observe?

Low-lying maxillary labial frenum.

The following teeth are clearly visible:
$$\frac{6\,e\,d\,c\,b\,1\,|\,1\,b\,c\,d}{6\,e\,d\,c\,2\,1\,|\,1\,2\,c\,d\,e\,6}$$
Mild lower labial segment crowding with mesiolingual rotations of $\overline{1|1}$; slight spacing distal of $\overline{2|2}$.
Upper median diastema with the crowns of $1|1$ flared distally.
Class III incisor relationship.

Crossbites $\dfrac{b\,|\,b}{c\,|\,c}$

What is the aetiology of the rotations of $\overline{1|1}$?

Incisor rotations are usually a manifestation of inherent crowding, in the arch, which is genetic in origin. The unspaced primary lower incisors reported by the child's mother are predictive of likely crowding of the permanent successors. Incisor rotations may also arise from ectopic position of the tooth germs or from the presence of a supernumerary tooth.

What are the possible causes of the upper median diastema?

These are listed in **Table 1.1**.

Table 1.1 Causes of an upper median diastema

Causes	Comments
Developmental	Due to pressure of 2‾2 on 1‾1 roots ('ugly duckling' stage); tends to resolve by the time 3‾3 erupt
Dentoalveolar disproportion	Small teeth in a large arch
Absent or peg-shaped 2s	
Supernumerary tooth/teeth in midline	
Proclination of 21‾12	May be due to digit sucking habit
Prominent labial frenum	Implicated where blanching of the incisive papilla exists on stretching the frenum and notching between 1‾1 exists on radiograph
Pathological	Cyst/tumour Juvenile periodontitis

Table 1.2 Eruption dates for primary and permanent teeth

Primary	Months	Permanent	Years
Upper		**Upper**	
Central incisor	6–7	Central incisor	7–8
Lateral incisor	7–8	Lateral incisor	8–9
Canine	18–20	Canine	11–12
First molar	12–15	First premolar	10–11
Second molar	24–36	Second premolar	10–12
		First molar	6–7
		Second molar	12–13
		Third molar	17–21
Lower		**Lower**	
Central incisor	6–7	Central incisor	6–7
Lateral incisor	7–8	Lateral incisor	7–8
Canine	18–20	Canine	9–10
First molar	12–15	First premolar	10–12
Second molar	24–36	Second premolar	11–12
		First molar	5–6
		Second molar	12–13
		Third molar	17–21

Is the dental and occlusal development normal?

Dental development is normal. Eruption dates of the primary and permanent dentition are given in **Table 1.2**.

It is common for some crowding to be present as the lower incisors erupt, which usually manifests itself as slight lingual placement and/or rotation of the teeth, but the slight distal tilt and rotations of $\overline{1|1}$ may indicate inherent crowding. There is also no lower primate space visible between the primary canines and first primary molars.

Spacing between the upper permanent central incisors (flared distally and known as the 'ugly duckling' stage) is also normal at this stage, but generalized spacing of the upper primary teeth including the upper primate spaces (located between the upper primary lateral incisors and the upper primary canines) should exist.

Although the primary incisor relationship is commonly edge-to-edge at 5–6 years with incisor attrition, it is not usual for the permanent incisor relationship to be similar. Rather a Class I incisor relationship should be present.

A crossbite should not exist on $\dfrac{b|b}{c|c}$

The first permanent molars should normally be in half-unit Class II relationship due to the 'flush terminal planes' relationship of the second primary molars.

Key point

On eruption:
- Some crowding of $\overline{21|12}$ is usual.
- A median diastema between 1|1 is normal.

How is space created for the upper permanent incisor teeth?

Space is obtained from three sources: the spacing which should exist between the primary incisors; an increase in intercanine width; and by the permanent upper incisors erupting more proclined and labial to their predecessors.

Investigation
What investigations would you undertake? Explain why
- **Clinical**

Gently pull the upper lip upwards and observe if there is blanching of the incisive papilla from the frenal attachment. This may implicate the frenum in the possible aetiology of the upper median diastema. Slight blanching of the incisive papilla was detected.

Check if there is a mandibular displacement associated with the crossbites on $\dfrac{b|b}{c|c}$. If a displacement is detected, early crossbite correction is indicated. However, in this case no displacement existed and this is confirmed by the absence of a lower centreline shift.

- **Radiographic**

    A dental panoramic tomogram is required to ascertain the presence, position and form of all unerupted teeth.

    If a supernumerary tooth/teeth or other pathology is observed or suspected on the dental panoramic tomogram in the anterior premaxilla, a standard occlusal radiograph should be taken.

The dental panoramic tomogram is shown in Figure 1.3. What do you notice?

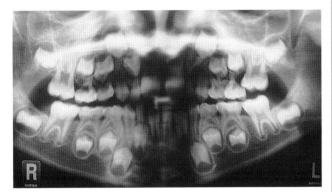

Fig. 1.3 Dental panoramic tomogram.

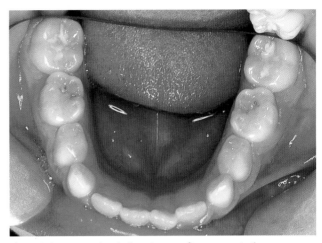

Fig. 1.4 Lower occlusal view 1 year after presentation.

Normal alveolar bone levels.

A normally developing dentition, which is consistent with the patient's chronological age.

Resorption of the distal root of $\underline{e|e}$.

Impaction of $\underline{|6}$.

Diagnosis
What is the diagnosis?

Mild Class III malocclusion in the early mixed dentition on a Class I skeletal base with average FMPA. Mild lower labial segment crowding; upper median diastema. Crossbite $\dfrac{b|b}{c|c}$ with no mandibular displacement. Impacted $\underline{|6}$.

What treatment would you advise for the labial segment problems? Explain why

No treatment is indicated at present. The mild lower labial segment crowding may reduce slightly by drift of $\overline{2|2}$ into the small existing spaces distal to them (**Fig. 1.4**). There is also likely to be some increase in lower intercanine width until about 9 years of age, which may reduce the lower incisor crowding further.

The upper median diastema is likely to reduce as the maxillary permanent lateral incisors and canines erupt. Brian's mother should be reassured about this. The attachment of the maxillary labial frenum, although initially to the incisive papilla during the primary dentition, moves to the palatal aspect as the permanent lateral incisors erupt and approximate the permanent central incisors (**Fig. 1.5**). In a spaced arch, this migration of the frenum is less likely. In contrast, where the upper arch is potentially crowded and the diastema is less than 4 mm, recession of the frenum and closure of the median diastema may be forthcoming eventually. How-ever, as Brian's father had an upper median diastema, there may be a tendency for the space to persist.

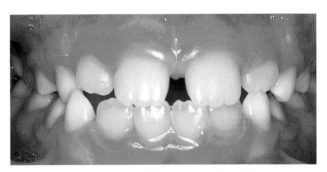

Fig. 1.5 Anterior occlusion following eruption of $\underline{2}$'s.

What is the prevalence of impacted $\underline{6}$'s?

The prevalence of this eruption disturbance varies between 2% and 6%, although in children with cleft lip and/or palate, a 20–25% prevalence has been reported.

What are the causes of impaction of $\underline{6}$'s?

Impaction of $\underline{6}$ is indicative of crowding.

Both local and hereditary factors have been reported (**Table 1.3**). A multifactorial mode of inheritance has been identified where both genetic and local factors can act in combination.

Table 1.3 Causes of impaction (ectopic eruption) of $\underline{6}$'s

Factor	Cause
Local	Significantly larger $\underline{6}$'s and more pronounced mesial angle of eruption of $\underline{6}$'s
Hereditary	Familial tendency Small maxilla

Describe the clinical features of ectopic eruption of $\underline{6}$ and classification of this anomaly

Ectopic eruption of $\underline{6}$ is manifested by eruption mesial of its normal path. Complete eruption of $\underline{6}$ is initially blocked by the distal surface of e, which then, in response to tooth contact, undergoes resorption.

Ectopic eruption of 6 is described as 'reversible' if disimpaction and full eruption ensue spontaneously. After 8 years of age, this occurs rarely. If 6 remains impacted until treated or premature loss of e happens spontaneously, ectopic eruption of 6 is described as 'irreversible'.

Treatment
What treatment options are there for irreversible ectopic eruption of 6'?
● **Without extraction of e**

A brass wire separator may be tightened around the contact area of e and 6 over several visits. Discing the distal surface of e or the use of a separating spring have been proposed also.

If 6 exhibits marked mesial tipping, more active distal movement is required. This may be achieved by a spring, soldered to a transpalatal bar uniting d's. The spring acts against a composite stop bonded to the occlusal surface of 6.

● **With extraction of e**

If there is marked resorption or abscess formation of e, or if 6 cannot be disimpacted with a separating spring, or if 6 is carious and poor access impedes restoration, extraction of e is unavoidable. As 6 erupts with a mesial inclination, space loss occurs rapidly following loss of e. Consideration should be given to regaining space by distalizing 6 with a spring on an upper removable appliance in cases of unilateral loss of e. Where bilateral loss of e occurs, distal movement of 6's may be achieved by springs soldered to a transpalatal arch connecting both d's or by cervical traction to bands on 6's. Alternatively, management of the space loss resulting from extraction of e's can be deferred until the permanent dentition.

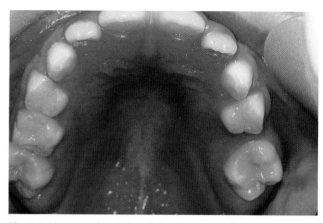

Fig. 1.6 Upper occlusal view following extraction of |e .

How will the orthodontist manage impaction of |6 in this case?

The various options regarding disimpaction of 6's should be discussed with Brian and his parents.

It should then be explained that if |e becomes abscessed, or attempts to disimpact |6 are unsuccessful, extraction of |e will be required. Treatment to deal with the resultant space loss will be required thereafter.

Brian was not keen for any orthodontic treatment and, therefore, it was decided to extract |e in view of the caries risk to |6 . The consequent upper buccal segment crowding (**Fig. 1.6**) will be dealt with in the permanent dentition.

Impressions and a wax registration for study models should be recorded of the developing Class III malocclusion, which should then be monitored until the permanent dentition is fully established, when treatment planning can be completed.

Recommended reading
Foster TD, Grundy MC 1986 Occlusal changes from primary to permanent dentitions. Br J Orthod 13:187–193.

Huang WJ, Creath CJ 1995 The midline diastema: a review of its aetiology and treatment. Pediatr Dent 17:171–179.

Kurol J, Bjerklin K 1986 Ectopic eruption of maxillary first permanent molars: a review. ASDC J Dent Child 53:209–214.

For revision see Mind Maps 1a and 1b, pages 146–147

Key point
For impacted 6 consider:
● Brass wire separator.
● Disc distal surface of e.
● Move 6 distally.
● Extract e.

2

Unerupted upper central incisor

Summary

Neil, a 9-year-old boy, presents with 1| unerupted (**Fig. 2.1**). What are the possible causes and how would you manage the problem?

History

● Complaint

Neil's mother is very concerned about the unerupted 1| as he is 9 years old and the tooth has not yet appeared. 2| is also erupting over b| and she dislikes the appearance.

● History of complaint

|a was lost at about 6 years and |1 erupted normally at 6.5 years. Unfortunately, Neil fell over in the school yard 4 months ago and fractured |1, exposing the pulp, which was subsequently extirpated. For the present, the root canal of |1 has been filled with non-setting calcium hydroxide

Is there anything else you would wish to elicit from the history?

Neil's mother should be asked about any history of trauma to the primary incisors, particularly intrusion of ba|.

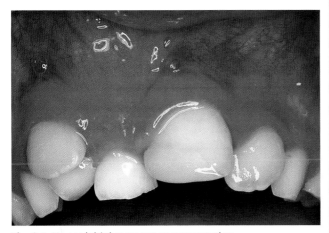

Fig. 2.1 Upper labial segment at presentation.

There is no history of trauma to the primary dentition.

● Medical history

Neil is fit and well.

Examination

● Extra-oral examination

Neil has a mild Class II skeletal pattern with slightly increased FMPA. His lips are competent. No facial asymmetry or abnormal temporomandibular joint signs or symptoms were detected.

● Intra-oral examination

The appearance of the mouth is shown in Figures 2.1 and 2.2. What do you notice?

Oral hygiene is fair—calculus is visible on the buccal aspect of 6|.

Mild plaque deposits on most teeth associated with marginal gingival erythema.

Early mixed dentition with $\dfrac{6\,e\,d\,c\,2\,b\,a \mid 1\,2\,c\,d\,e\,6}{6\,e\,d\,c\,2\,1 \mid 1\,2\,c\,e\,6}$ present.

Restored incisal edge of |1.

Class I malocclusion with mild lower and moderate upper labial segment crowding.

Upper centreline to the right; lower centreline to the left.

Potential crowding lower left quadrant.

Buccal segment relationship Class I bilaterally.

Why are the centrelines displaced?

An imbalance of upper anterior tooth size (the retained a| is considerably smaller than an 1) has promoted the upper centreline shift but this has been aggravated by inherent upper arch crowding.

The lower centreline shift is due to early unbalanced loss of |d in a potentially crowded arch.

Could the lower centreline shift have been prevented?

Following removal of |d, the lower centreline should have been monitored at review visits. |d should have been extracted to balance for loss of |d when the centreline appeared to be migrating.

What are the possible causes of the unerupted 1|?

These are listed in **Box 2.1**.

> **Box 2.1** Causes of unerupted or missing upper permanent central incisor
>
> **Missing:**
> Congenitally absent
> Avulsed
> Extracted
>
> **Present but unerupted:**
> Ectopic position of the tooth germ
> Dilaceration and/or displacement due to trauma
> Scar tissue
> Supernumerary tooth
> Crowding
> Pathology e.g. cyst, odontogenic tumour

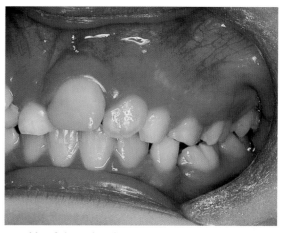

Fig. 2.2 (c) Left buccal occlusion.

How would you rate the likelihood in this case of each of the potential causes of unerupted 1| listed in Box 2.1?

Congenital absence of 1| is highly unlikely. It would be very rare for 1| to be absent without other congenitally missing teeth.

Avulsion of 1| can be excluded as there is no history of 1| having erupted or of incisor trauma.

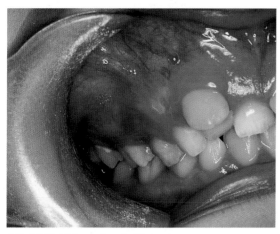

Fig. 2.2 (a) Right buccal occlusion.

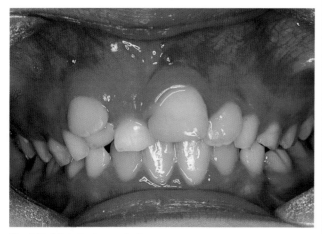

Fig. 2.2 (b) Anterior occlusion.

> **Box 2.2** Classification of supernumerary teeth by morphology
>
> ● Conical or peg-shaped—most often lies between 1|1 and may produce no effect, a median diastema, incisor rotation or failure of 1 eruption
> ● Tuberculate or barrel-shaped—most usually associated with unerupted 1
> ● Supplemental—resembles and lies adjacent to the last tooth of a series (2's, 5's, 8's)
> ● Odontome—may either be compound or complex

Extraction of 1| can be excluded also.

Ectopic position of the tooth germ is a possibility but is more likely to be secondary to some pathological cause or the presence of a supernumerary tooth.

Dilaceration and/or displacement due to trauma can be excluded due to the absence of a relevant history.

Scar tissue can be excluded also as this would result from trauma.

A supernumerary tooth (**Box 2.2**) is the most likely cause of unerupted 1| . With an incidence of 1–3% in the premaxilla, supernumerary teeth (particularly the late-forming tuberculate type) are associated with delay or non-eruption of an upper permanent central incisor.

Crowding is an unlikely cause. Although the upper labial segment is crowded, only very severe crowding would prevent 1| erupting, 2 years following its expected eruption time.

Pathology is also an unlikely cause. There is no evidence of alveolar expansion in the premaxilla, which would most likely be due to cyst formation possibly arising from 1| , a supernumerary or odontome. Other rarer lesions would need to be excluded.

Key point

● A supernumerary tooth is the most common cause of failure of eruption of 1.

Investigation

What investigations are required? Explain why

● **Clinical**

Palpation of the labial and palatal mucosae in the 1| area to detect if the unerupted 1| is present.

● **Radiographic**

The following views are required to determine the presence/absence of 1| , and/or possible supernumerary teeth:

Dental panoramic tomogram gives a general screen of the developing dentition allowing detection of the presence/absence of unerupted teeth.

Standard occlusal or periapical views provide greater detail of the anterior maxilla. In particular, the crown and root morphology of unerupted 1| , the presence of supernumerary teeth and/or other pathology and their relation to the incisor roots as well as the root and periapical status of traumatized |1 can be assessed. On a panoramic radiograph these structures may be poorly defined due to super-imposition of other anatomical features or by lying outside the focal trough of the tomogram.

Periapical radiographs should include the roots of adjacent teeth to determine if they were damaged during previous trauma to |1 .

Used in combination and employing the principle of vertical parallax, the dental panoramic tomogram and the standard occlusal or periapical views can be used to localize the position of any unerupted tooth and/or supernumerary relative to the dental arch.

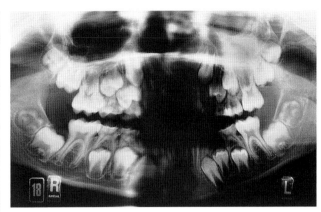

Fig. 2.3 (a) Dental panoramic tomogram.

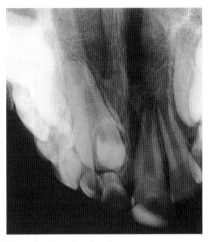

Fig. 2.3 (b) Standard occlusal radiograph.

Key point

● Two radiographic views are required to localize an unerupted tooth in the premaxilla using parallax.

A *lateral view* may be required to aid localization of a dilaceration, if visible on either the dental panoramic tomogram or on the standard occlusal/periapical views.

How would you determine the position of an unerupted tooth in the anterior premaxilla using vertical parallax?

If the tooth moves in the same direction as the tube shift, it lies palatal to the arch; if it moves in the opposite direction to the tube shift, it lies buccal to the arch. Where there is no apparent shift in its position between the films, it lies in the line of the arch.

Neil's radiographs are shown in Figure 2.3. *What do these show?*

The panoramic tomograph shows all permanent teeth to be present including third molars. Dental development appears reasonably aligned with chronological age. There is a supernumerary tooth overlying 1| . Root resorption of the remaining first primary molars is advanced and caries is evident in $\frac{d|}{e\,d\,|\,e}$. Bitewing radiography would be required for more accurate assessment of the extent of carious involvement of the primary molars.

The standard occlusal view shows that root resorption of ba| is advanced. 1| has a normal crown and root form, the root canal appears wide with an apical calcific bridge. A tuberculate supernumerary overlies the crown of 1| . The composite tip repair to |1 is visible and its apex is incomplete but narrowing.

Application of vertical parallax to these radiographs indicates that 1| and the supernumerary tooth are palatally positioned.

Diagnosis

What is your diagnosis?

Class I malocclusion on a mild Class II skeletal base with slightly increased FMPA.

Generalized mild marginal gingivitis.

Caries in $\frac{d|}{e\,d\,|\,e}$; |1 traumatized and restored.

Upper and lower arch crowding.

ba| retained; 2| erupting labially; 1| erupted with associated tuberculate supernumerary.

Upper centreline shift to the right; lower centreline shift to the left.

Buccal segment relationship Class I bilaterally.

What is the IOTN DHC score? (see p. 183) Explain why

5i due to impeded eruption of 1| caused by the presence of a supernumerary tooth.

Treatment
What are your aims of treatment?

Restore gingival and dental health.

Relief of crowding.

Correction of centrelines.

Alignment of 1| .

What is your treatment plan?

1. Oral hygiene instruction.
2. Dietary advice with the aid of a diet diary.
3. Determine the prognosis of the second primary molars from bitewing radiographs.

e's were deemed to be of reasonable prognosis but ē's require formocresol pulpotomy and stainless steel crowns or extraction in view of the pulpal carious involvement. More than half the root length of e|e remains and in view of the space loss that already exists in the lower arch, it would be wise to minimize any further extractions except in an attempt to correct the centreline shift.

4. Fit an upper removable appliance to open space for 1| and correct the upper centreline.

5. Taking the poor prognosis of $\frac{d|}{d|}$ into account, and to allow relief of upper arch crowding at this stage, to create space for centreline correction and for 1| to be accommodated, the following extractions are indicated $\frac{d\ c\ a\ |\ b\ c\ d}{d\ |}$

   Removal of |d is required to balance the extraction of d| . Extraction of d̄| will balance the loss of |d̄ and tend to encourage correction of the lower centreline shift.

6. The supernumerary tooth will also need to be surgically removed and an attachment with a length of gold chain should be bonded to 1| followed by flap replacement (closed technique). 1| should not be surgically exposed.

7. In this case it will be necessary to await full eruption of 2| , following removal of ba| , before moving it distally to create space for 1| .

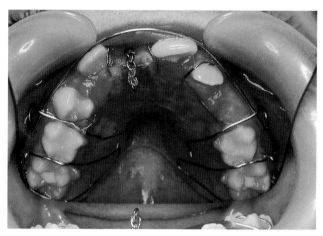

Fig. 2.4 Upper removable appliance to open space for 1| .

What design of upper removable appliance would you use to achieve the desired tooth movements?

Palatal finger springs (0.5 mm stainless steel wire) to 2|12 .

Adams clasps (0.7 mm stainless steel wire) to 6|6 .

Recurved labial bow (0.7 mm stainless steel wire).

Full palatal acrylic coverage (**Fig. 2.4**).

When space for 1| has been created, a hook may be soldered to the labial bow to allow attachment of the gold chain for 1| extrusion or the bow may be modified to create a buccal arm for this purpose.

Will an upper removable appliance achieve all the treatment objectives?

An upper removable appliance will achieve the simple tooth movements (tipping and extrusion) required in this case at this stage. It is likely that further treatment, probably loss of a premolar unit from each quadrant and fixed appliance therapy, will be required at a later date and detailing of 1| position can be undertaken at that stage.

How would you ensure long-term stability of 1| following alignment?

Bonded palatal retention will be required to guarantee long-term alignment of 1| .

Labial gingivoplasty may be required at a later stage in relation to 1| to obtain coincidence of the gingival margins of 1|1 .

Key point

Sequence in management of unerupted 1:
- Open space for unerupted 1.
- Remove supernumerary.
- Bond attachment to 1.
- Do not surgically expose 1.
- Align 1 with appropriate appliance.
- Maintain 1 correction with bonded retainer.

Recommended reading

Becker A, Brin I, Ben-Bassat Y, Zilberman Y, Chaushu S 2002 Closed eruption surgical technique for impacted maxillary incisors: a post orthodontic periodontal evaluation. Am J Orthod Dentofacial Orthop 22:9–14.

Burden D, Harper C, Mitchell L, Mitchell N, Richmond S 1997 The management of unerupted maxillary incisors. National Clinical Guidelines (Orthodontics), Faculty of Dental Surgery. Available: www.rcseng.ac.uk/dental/fds/clinical_guidelines 1997

For revision see Mind Map 2, page 148

3

Absent upper lateral incisors

Summary

Sarah, aged 12, presents with spacing of her upper anterior teeth (**Fig. 3.1**). What are the possible causes and how may it be treated?

History

● Complaint

Sarah does not like the gaps between her upper front teeth. She has just moved to a new school and feels self-conscious about the appearance of her teeth.

● History of complaint

All primary teeth were present and were lost normally. When her upper permanent front teeth erupted, there was considerable spacing between them and this has not altered much since then. The permanent teeth erupted at a normal age and none have been extracted or avulsed.

● Medical history

Sarah is fit and well.

● Dental history

Sarah attends her general dental practitioner regularly but has had no intervention other than placement of fissure sealants to first permanent molars.

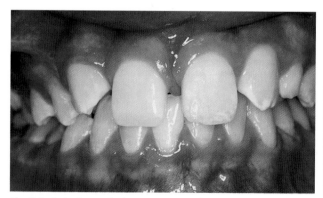

Fig. 3.1 Anterior occlusion at presentation.

● Family history

Sarah's mother also has a small space between her upper front teeth due to one missing tooth ($\underline{2|}$).

Social history

Sarah is a keen flautist and not motivated to wearing a fixed appliance.

Examination

● Extraoral

Sarah has a Class I skeletal pattern with average FMPA; there is no facial asymmetry. Her lips are competent with the lower lip covering the incisal third of the upper incisors. The temporomandibular joints are symptom-free.

What else should you check for?

Thinning of the hair.
Absence of palmar sweat glands.
These signs are present in anhydrotic ectodermal dysplasia, which is associated with marked hypodontia (see Chapter 32).

● Intraoral

The intraoral views are shown in Figures 3.1 *and 3.2. What do these show?*

The soft tissues appear healthy and overall oral hygiene seems good, although there are small plaque deposits labially on the lower incisors. All teeth are of good quality and no caries is evident.
The following teeth are present:

$$\frac{7\ 6\ 5\ 4\ 3\ 1\ \ |1\ 3\ c\ 4\ 5\ 6\ 7}{7\ 6\ 5\ 4\ 3\ 2\ 1|1\ 2\ 3\ 4\ 5\ 6\ 7}$$

There is a retained fragment of $\overline{e|}$.
There is mild imbrication of the lower incisors, the upper arch is spaced.
The incisor relationship is Class I with a complete overbite.
The lower centreline is shifted slightly to the left.
The buccal segment relationship is half unit Class II bilaterally.

What other clinic assessment would you undertake?

The labial and palatal mucosa in the $\underline{2}$ area should be palpated for the presence of an unerupted tooth or any pathology.

What are the possible causes of the upper labial segment spacing?

These are listed in **Table 3.1**.

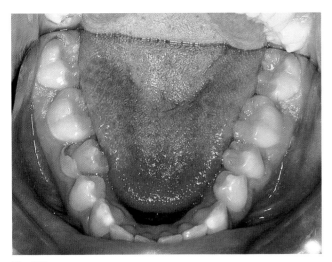

Fig. 3.2 a

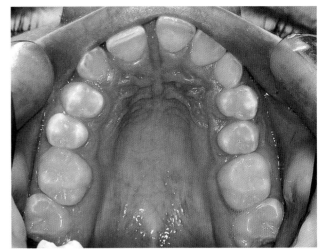

Fig. 3.2 b

Fig. 3.2 c

Fig. 3.2 d

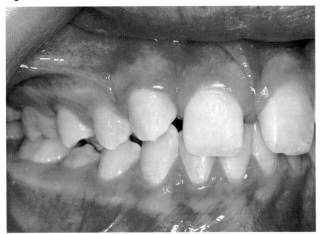

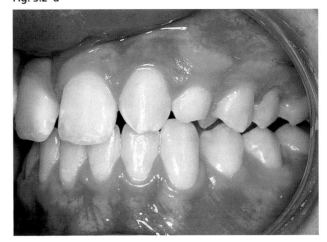

Fig. 3.2 (a) Lower occlusal view. (b) Upper occlusal view. (c) Right buccal occlusion. (d) Left buccal occlusion.

Table 3.1 Possible causes of the upper labial segment spacing

Cause	Aetiology
Absence of 2|2	Hypodontia (affects ~2% of Caucasians)—also associated with cleft lip and palate, Down syndrome and ectodermal dysplasia
	Avulsion
	Extraction
Failure of/delayed eruption of 2's	Crowding
	Ectopic position
	Supernumerary tooth
	Scar tissue
	Dilaceration
	Cyst/tumour

What is the most likely cause in this case?

Congenital absence of 2\|2 is most likely. This is more common in females than males. The genetic linkage is indicated by Sarah's mother, who has absence of 2\|.

Key point

● Congenital absence of 2's is more common in females.

What further investigations would you undertake?

● **Clinical**

Sensibility testing of the upper incisor and canine teeth is necessary to ensure their pulpal status is sound.

● **Radiographic**

A dental panoramic tomogram is required to determine the presence/absence of 2's, 8's, supernumerary teeth or any pathology.

● **Occlusal**

Impressions and a wax registration should be taken for study models to allow further assessment of the occlusion. Sarah's dental panoramic tomogram showed:

Normal alveolar bone height.
Absence of 2|2 and third molars; short root to |c .
No pathology associated with any erupted or
unerupted teeth.

What is your diagnosis?

Class I malocclusion on a Class I skeletal base with
average FMPA. Well-cared-for mouth. Uncrowded lower
arch; spaced upper arch with absent 2|2 . Buccal
segment relationship is half-unit Class II bilaterally.

What is the IOTN DHC grade (see p. 183)?

4h due to absence of 2|2 .

What are the treatment options?

These are:
1. Accept the spacing—not a realistic option as
   Sarah is concerned by it.
2. Build up the mediodistal width of 1's and 3's with
   composite or by veneering to reduce the spacing
   but not to close it completely. The median diastema
   is too large for restorative build up of 1|1 to look
   aesthetic. Some recontouring of the cusp tips of
   3's would also be required to improve the final
   appearance.
3. Orthodontic space closure. This would have
   required a considerable amount of tooth
   movement along with |c extraction and the
   wearing of a fixed appliance and reverse headgear.
4. Orthodontic space opening (this would require
   extraction of |c) for replacement of 2's on resin-
   retained bridges, by fixed bridgework or by
   implants in late teenage years. Replacement of 2's
   by autotransplantation of lower premolars is not a
   viable consideration as: (i) the lower arch does not
   warrant premolar extractions; and (ii) root
   formation on lower premolars is in advance of the
   ideal stage.

As option 2 will only partly address Sarah's concerns
it has to be ruled out. The choice then is between the two
orthodontic options.

Key point

Management options with absent 2's are to:
● Maintain or close 2 space.
● Open space for 2 replacement.

What factors would you consider in deciding between space closure or space opening?

Sarah should be seen with a restorative colleague who
will provide input regarding the restorative implications
of each treatment option. Then, it is often wise to
undertake a trial set-up of the optimal treatment option
using duplicate study models.

The following factors should be considered:
The patient's attitude to orthodontic treatment. If the
   patient is not keen on wearing fixed appliances,
   this may necessitate a change in treatment plan.
The anteroposterior and vertical skeletal relationships. In
   Class II cases with an increased overjet, space
   closure is desirable as it will eliminate the overjet,
   whereas in Class III cases this would tend to
   worsen the incisor relationship. Space opening is
   optimal in Class III cases where proclination of the
   incisors is likely to correct an anterior crossbite.
   Where the FMPA is reduced, space opening is
   preferable to space closure and the converse is true
   where an increased FMPA exists.
*The colour, size, shape and inclination of the canine and
   incisor teeth.* Where the maxillary canine is
   considerably darker than the incisors and/or it has
   a marked canine form, space closure is not
   advisable as considerable recontouring of 3's will
   be required to enable them to resemble 2's. Where
   the canine and incisor teeth are so inclined that it
   is possible to reposition them into their desired
   locations by tipping movements, a removable
   rather than a fixed appliance may be used.
*Whether the arches are spaced or crowded, and the buccal
   segment occlusion.* In uncrowded or mildly crowded
   arches, where the buccal segment occlusion is
   Class I or at most half-unit Class II, space opening
   is best. Space closure is preferable where crowding
   exists and the buccal segment relationship is a full-
   unit Class II.

In this case, it was decided to proceed with space opening
for replacement of 2|2, ultimately on resin-retained
bridges. This required an initial phase of distal movement
of the upper buccal segments to achieve a Class I molar
relationship, followed by retraction of 3's to a Class I
relationship with 3̄'s and space opening for 2's
replacement. Importantly, overbite reduction was also
undertaken in conjunction with these tooth movements
to provide space for the metal framework of the resin-
retained bridges.

Ideally, a fixed appliance would be indicated to achieve
these objectives, but as Sarah was not keen for this form
of treatment, an acceptable though not optimal outcome
was deemed achievable by upper removable appliance
therapy.

Key point

With absent 2's consider:
● Patient's attitude to orthodontic treatment.
● Skeletal relationships.
● Colour, size, shape and inclination of 3 and 1.
● Crowding/spacing.
● Buccal segment occlusion.

How could the upper buccal segments be moved distally using a removable appliance to achieve a Class I molar relationship?

An upper removable appliance with bilateral screws to move 6 5 4| and |4 5 6 distally is an option. Anchorage needs to be reinforced by allowing provision for headgear to be attached to the appliance. The appliance should also incorporate:

- Adams clasps (0.7 mm stainless steel wire) with headgear tubes soldered to 6's clasp bridges.
- Short labial bow 3| to |3.
- Flat anterior biteplane to half the crown height of 1|1 and extended 3 mm further palatally than the maximum overjet measurement.

When there is evidence of full-time appliance wear, headgear should be fitted for anchorage with an upward direction of pull to prevent the appliance becoming dislodged during headgear wear.

What force and duration of headgear wear is required for anchorage?

A force of 200–250 g per side for 10–12 hours per day is required.

What precautions must be adhered to when prescribing headgear?

Two safety mechanisms must be fitted to the headgear assembly, preferably a safety release spring mechanism attached to the headcap and a facebow with locking device. Verbal and written safety instructions must be issued to both patient and parents. The headgear should be checked at each visit.

When compliance with headgear wear is evident, then Sarah should be instructed to turn each screw once per week. |c should be extracted to allow for potential distal drift of |3 as the buccal segments are retracted to Class I. Some over-retraction is advisable to allow for any slight anchorage slip during the next phase of treatment when 3's will be retracted to a Class I relationship with 3̄'s, 1's will be approximated and overbite reduction will be maintained.

What design of upper removable appliance would you consider for these tooth movements?

Palatal finger springs to 3 1|1 3 (0.5 mm stainless steel wire).
Adams clasps 6|6 (0.7 mm stainless steel wire) with headgear tubes soldered to the clasp bridges.
Long labial bow with 'u' loops (0.7 mm stainless steel wire) from 4| to |4.

Flat anterior biteplane to half the crown height of 1|1 and extended 3 mm further palatally than the maximum overjet measurement. This is an important component of the appliance to ensure that overbite reduction is maintained, creating sufficient interocclusal clearance for placement of the metal framework on the resin-bonded bridges.

When space has been created for 2|2, what should be done?

The patient should be seen again with a restorative colleague to ensure that the tooth movements achieved will allow restorative treatment to proceed as planned. Then a removable retainer should be fitted for 6 months carrying replacement 2|2 and ensuring that space for them is maintained by placing wire spurs in contact with the adjoining teeth (**Fig. 3.3**).

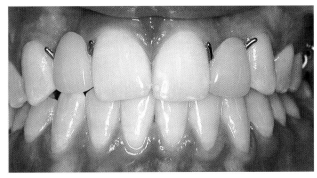

Fig. 3.3 Upper removable appliance retainer with replacement 2's.

Key point

- Always place wire spurs on the removable retainer, to the teeth adjoining the 2 space after space opening.

What design of resin-retained bridge is required?

Maintenance of closure of the median diastema requires permanent retention. A bonded palatal retainer framework linking 1|1 together is indicated along with resin-retained bridges with single wing, off 3|3. It is better that 1|1 are retained as a separate unit rather than risk the retention integrity and success of the bridges by incorporating 1|1 retention in the bridge design.

Implant replacement of 2|2 later is unlikely as the roots of 3 1|1 3 are tipped toward the 2|2 space, compromising access for implant positioning. The final result with 2|2 replaced on adhesive bridgework is shown in **Figure 3.4**.

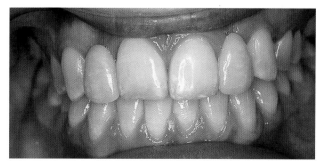

Fig. 3.4 Final restorations.

Recommended reading

Carter NE, Gillgrass TJ, Hobson RS, Jepson N, Meechan JG, Nohl FS, Nunn JH 2003 The interdisciplinary management of hypodontia: orthodontics. Br Dent J 194:361–366.

Harrison JE, Bowden DEJ 1992 The orthodontic/restorative interface. Restorative procedures to aid orthodontic treatment. Br J Orthod 19:143–152.

Mossey PA 1999 The heritability of malocclusion: part 2. The influence of genetics in malocclusion. Br J Orthod 26:195–203.

Robertsson S, Mohlin B 2000 The congenitally missing upper lateral incisor. A retrospective study of orthodontic space closure versus restorative treatment. Eur J Orthod 22:697–710.

For revision see Mind Map 3, page 149

4

Crowding and buccal upper canines

Summary

Gemma, an 11-year-old girl, attends for a 6-month dental assessment at your practice with both upper permanent canines erupting buccally (**Fig. 4.1**). What is the cause and how may it be treated?

History
● Complaint

Gemma does not like the 'squint' appearance of her top and bottom teeth, in particular the position of the upper eye teeth, which she says 'look like fangs'.

● History of complaint

The crookedness of Gemma's teeth has been getting worse for the past year. The appearance of her upper teeth has become of more concern to her in recent months when both upper eye teeth started to erupt. She is now teased at school and called 'Fangs', which annoys her.

Gemma's mother reports that her daughter's baby teeth were also slightly crooked. Both she and Gemma are very keen for treatment.

● Medical history

Gemma has suffered from asthma since she was 5 years old and uses a ventolin inhaler; otherwise she is fit and well.

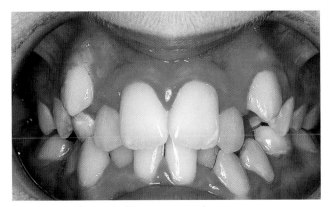

Fig. 4.1 Anterior occlusion at presentation.

● Dental history

Gemma has attended for routine dental examinations since she was 3 years old but has not undergone any active dental treatment.

Examination
● Extraoral

Gemma has a Class I skeletal pattern with average FMPA. There appears to be a slight facial asymmetry with the chin point deviated mildly to the right. The lips are competent.

No temporomandibular signs or symptoms were detected or reported.

Gemma and her mother were unaware of Gemma's slight facial asymmetry and noticed no change in her facial appearance over recent years.

Would you be concerned by the mild facial asymmetry?

A mild degree of facial asymmetry is normal and as facial appearance is reportedly unaltered for several years there is no cause for concern.

● Intraoral
Gemma's intraoral views are shown in Figures 4.1 and 4.2. What do you notice?

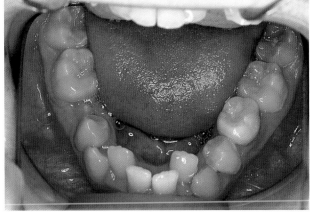

Fig. 4.2 (a) Lower occlusal view.

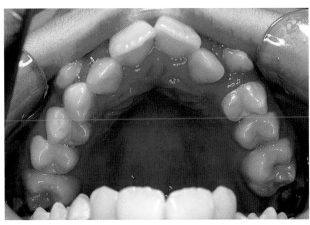

Fig. 4.2 (b) Upper occlusal view.

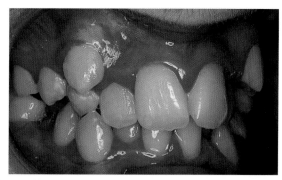

Fig. 4.2 (c) Right buccal occlusion.

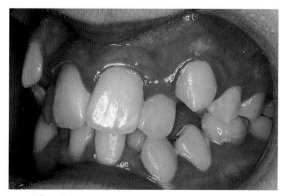

Fig. 4.2 (d) Left buccal occlusion.

Generalized marginal gingival erythema.

Plaque deposits visible on several teeth, notably both 3's.

There are no restorations and there is no obvious caries.

Gemma is in the late mixed dentition stage with the following teeth present: $\frac{6\,5\,4\,c\,3\,2\,1\,|\,1\,2\,3\,4\,5\,6}{7\,6\,5\,4\,3\,2\,1\,\,|\,1\,2\,3\,4\,e\,6\,7}$.

5⌐ and 7|7 are partially erupted.

The lower labial segment is moderately crowded with 2|2 bodily displaced lingually and 1|1 slightly mesiolabially rotated.

3⌐ is distally inclined; ⌐3 is mesially inclined.

The lower right buccal segment is also crowded with insufficient space for 5⌐ ; the lower left buccal segment is uncrowded with ⌐e present.

The upper labial segment is moderately crowded, with 1|1 slightly mesiolabially rotated and 3|3 erupting buccally; c| is present. 3| is upright and |3 is slightly distally inclined. The upper buccal segments are aligned.

In occlusion, there is a Class I incisor relationship.

The overbite is average and complete. The lower centreline is slightly to the right.

The right molar relationship is Class III and the left molar relationship is Class I.

What are the possible reasons for 3's erupting buccally?

Crowding—buccal displacement of 3's is often a manifestation of inherent crowding in the upper arch. A contributory factor is 3 being the last tooth to erupt anterior to the first permanent molars.

Retention of the primary canine—this usually leads to slight buccal displacement of 3.

Key point

● Buccal displacement of 3 is more usual in a crowded arch.

Investigations

What investigations would you request and why?

A dental panoramic tomogram is required to provide a general view of the developing dentition and confirm the presence and position of all unerupted permanent teeth.

Gemma's dental panoramic tomogram is shown in Figure 4.3. What do you notice?

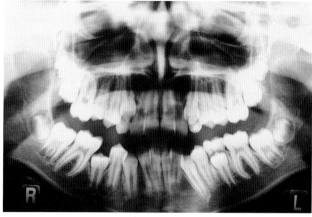

Fig. 4.3 Dental panoramic tomogram.

Alveolar bone level is normal.

Presence of a full complement of developing permanent teeth including third molars.

All teeth appear caries-free.

What is your diagnosis?

Class I malocclusion on a Class I skeletal base with average FMPA with the chin point displaced slightly to the right.

Generalized marginal gingivitis.

Moderate upper and lower arch crowding with the lower centreline displaced slightly to the right.

Right molar relationship is Class III; left molar relationship is Class I.

What is the IOTN DHC score and why (see p. 183)?

4d due to severe displacements of teeth, greater than 4 mm.

Treatment
What treatment is likely to be required in this case? Explain why

Extractions are required to relieve the moderate crowding. Fixed appliance therapy is indicated in view of the distal inclination of most canines, the rotations of the central incisors, the bodily lingual displacement of $\overline{2}$'s and the centreline shift.

What would you do now?

Explain to the patient the likely plan for correction of her malocclusion.

Arrange for several visits of oral hygiene instruction by the practice hygenist, and assuming that oral hygiene improves satisfactorily, then take upper and lower impressions and a wax registration for study models.

Arrange referral to an orthodontist and enclose the study models and dental panoramic tomogram.

Write a referral letter to the orthodontist (**Fig. 4.4**).

What aims of treatment do you think will be proposed by the orthodontist?

Relief of crowding.
Upper and lower arch alignment.

Practice address

Date

Dear

Re [patient's name, address, date of birth]

I would be grateful if you could see Gemma for orthodontic assessment and treatment.

Gemma's oral hygiene is improving following several visits to our hygenist. She has a caries-free dentition. She is very keen for treatment and is prepared to wear fixed appliances.

She has a Class I malocclusion on a Class I skeletal base with average FMPA and the chin point slightly to the right. The upper and lower arches are moderately crowded and the lower centreline is slightly to the right.

I enclose current study models and a recent dental panoramic tomogram.

Yours sincerely

Fig. 4.4 Example of a referral letter.

Correction of lower centreline.
Correction of right molar relationship.
Closure of any residual spacing.

Describe how you would approach treatment planning

1. *Consider the lower arch first and plan the lower labial segment.* As the latter is in a narrow zone of soft tissue balance between the lips and the tongue it is best to consider this sacrosanct. First the alignment of the labial segment must be assessed and if it is crowded, as in Gemma's case, the degree of crowding must be assessed to ascertain if this is sufficient to warrant extractions.

As Gemma has moderate lower labial segment crowding, space will be required to achieve alignment.

What possible means are there of creating space?

Extractions.
Arch expansion.
Distal movement of the molars.
Enamel stripping.
Any combination of the above.

Expansion of the lower intercanine width is unstable, and distal movement of the lower first permanent molars is difficult without extraction of lower second permanent molars and is undertaken rarely. Enamel stripping is usually only considered in adults to gain 1–2 mm of space in total. In view of these considerations, extractions are the only realistic option of gaining space in Gemma's case.

Key point

● Always consider the lower arch first in treatment planning.

What factors govern the choice of extraction?

The prognosis of teeth.
The site of crowding.
The degree of crowding.
Individual tooth position, e.g. grossly displaced or ectopic teeth.

In this case, there are no lower teeth of poor prognosis and in view of the site and degree of crowding, lower first premolars would be the teeth of choice for extraction.

Why are first premolars a common choice of extraction?

They are in the middle of the arch and, therefore, provide space for relief of moderate labial and buccal segment crowding.

The contact point between the canine and second premolar is as good as between the canine and first premolar.

If the canine is mesially inclined, considerable scope exists for spontaneous alignment of the labial segment as the canine uprights into the extraction space. For maximum spontaneous improvement, it is best to extract the first premolars as the permanent canines are erupting.

Any residual space is not at the front of the mouth and is likely to close further with mesial drift of the buccal segments.

2. *Imagine the corrected position of* $\overline{3}$. $\overline{|3}$ is mesially inclined and will upright spontaneously following removal of $\overline{|4}$, thereby providing space for labial segment alignment; $\overline{3|}$, however, is distally inclined and will require bodily retraction with a fixed appliance.

3. *Mentally reposition* $\underline{3}$ *to be in a Class I relationship with the corrected position of* $\overline{3}$. Space is required in Gemma's case for this. Extraction of both upper first premolars should provide adequate space for retraction of $\underline{3}$'s. As $\underline{3|}$ is upright and $\underline{|3}$ is distally inclined, fixed appliance therapy is indicated to effect this movement.

4. *Plan the upper labial segment.* As the incisors are mildly crowded and slightly rotated, fixed appliance therapy is required to produce ideal alignment.

5. *Decide on the final molar relationship.* As upper and lower first premolar extractions are planned, the final molar relationship should be Class I. Closure of residual buccal segment spacing following the extractions will require fixed appliance therapy.

6. *Assess the anchorage needs.* As almost all of the upper first premolar extraction spaces will be required for relief of upper arch crowding, and retraction of the upright/distally inclined $\underline{3}$'s is needed, anchorage would be best reinforced with a palatal arch, attached to bands on $\underline{6}$'s.

7. *Plan retention.* The prognosis is favourable, but bonded retention to the lower labial segment would be wise in view of the bodily lingual displacement of $\overline{2|2}$. Upper removable retention for at least 12 months (6 months full-time except meals, followed by 6 months at night only) should be planned.

Key point

- Always plan anchorage at the treatment planning stage.
- The amount of space and type of intended tooth movement influence anchorage demands.
- Always consider retention in the treatment plan.

What is the final orthodontic treatment plan likely to be?

No appliance therapy would be considered until Gemma has demonstrated that she is capable of maintaining a high standard of oral hygiene. Then the orthodontic plan would be:

Extraction of four first premolars.

Upper and lower fixed appliance therapy with a palatal arch. (The palatal arch should be placed and Gemma's cooperation assessed before any extractions are requested.)

Upper removable retainer and lower bonded canine to canine retainer.

What risks should the patient be warned of regarding fixed appliance orthodontic treatment?

The patient should be warned of the risk of:
 Decalcification.
 Root resorption.
 Loss of tooth vitality.
 Relapse.

Gemma's final occlusion is shown in Figure 4.5. What undesirable sequelae of treatment are visible?

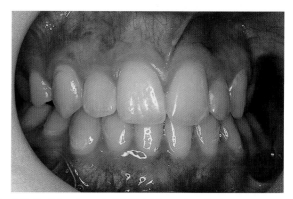

Fig. 4.5 Post-treatment. (a) Right buccal occlusion.

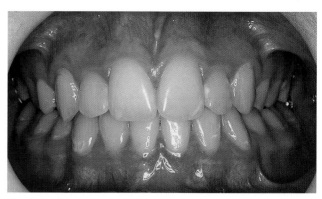

Fig. 4.5 (b) Anterior occlusion.

Several teeth are affected by white spot lesions or decalcification, indicating early carious involvement.

How common is this with fixed appliance therapy and which teeth are affected mostly?

The reported incidence is 2–96%. Upper lateral incisors and lower canines are affected most commonly.

How may the problem be prevented or minimized?

Careful patient selection. Ensure a high standard of oral hygiene pre-treatment.

Advise the patient that fizzy drinks and sugary foods should not be consumed between meals.

The teeth should be brushed with a fluoridated dentifrice after each meal.

Regular surveillance of oral hygiene and oral hygiene instruction should be undertaken by a hygenist throughout treatment.

Daily use of a fluoride mouthrinse (0.05% sodium fluoride) is recommended during treatment.

How may these 'white spots' be managed?

Usually, following removal of the appliances, they regress slightly as maintenance of an improved standard of oral hygiene is facilitated.

Application of high concentration fluoride varnish is inadvisable as this leads to hypermineralization of the white spot, which makes it more visible and less likely to regress.

Where the white spot lesions are extensive and pose an obvious aesthetic insult, acid–pumice abrasion with 0.2% hydrofluoric acid may be carried out. In severe cases, veneers or composite restorations are likely to be required.

Key point

Decalcification with fixed appliances
- Is common (2–96% incidence).
- Affects 2's and 3's mostly.
- Is best prevented by careful patient selection, dietary advice, use of fluoride mouthrinse.

Recommended reading

Benson PE, Parkin N, Millett DT et al 2004 Fluorides for the prevention of white spots on teeth during fixed brace treatment (Cochrane Review). In: The Cochrane Library Issue 3 John Wiley, Chichester.

Little RM, Wallen TR, Reidel RA 1981 Stability and relapse of mandibular anterior alignment-first premolar extraction cases treated by traditional edgewise orthodontics. Am J Orthod 80:349–65.

Mitchell L 1992 Decalcification during orthodontic treatment with fixed appliances: an overview. Br J Orthod 19:199–205.

Stephens CD 1989 The use of natural spontaneous tooth movement in the treatment of malocclusion. Dent Update 16:337–342.

For revision see Mind Map 4, page 150

Summary

Diane, a 15-year-old girl, presents with both upper primary canines retained (**Fig. 5.1**). What is the cause and what treatment possibilities are there?

History

Diane is concerned about the size of the baby upper 'eye' teeth that are present and by the spaces on either side of her upper two front teeth. She is not bothered by the small space between the upper front teeth. c| is also slightly loose and she is worried in case it is lost, producing a big space.

● History of complaint

Diane has been aware that the baby eye teeth should have been lost a few years ago. Her previous general dental practitioner, who retired last year, advised her that these teeth would eventually fall out by themselves and that when the new eye teeth came through, she would then need a brace to close the spaces between her top teeth. There is no history of trauma to c|c areas and all other primary teeth were lost naturally. All permanent teeth have erupted on schedule.

She has noticed that c| has been loose intermittently for the past 18 months. It does not appear to have got looser in recent months. Diane is very keen to improve the appearance of her upper teeth.

● Medical history

Diane is fit and well.

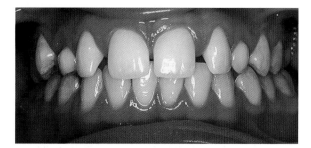

Fig. 5.1 Anterior occlusion at presentation.

● Dental history

Diane is a regular attender at her general dental practitioner but has never had any dental treatment.

Examination
● Extraoral

Diane has a Class I skeletal pattern with average FMPA and lower facial height and no facial asymmetry. Her lips are competent with the lower lip at the level of the incisal third of the upper incisors.

There is a slight lateral mandibular displacement to the left on closure on $\frac{4|}{4|}$.

● Intraoral

The intraoral views are shown in **Figures 5.1** *and* **5.2.** *Describe what you see*

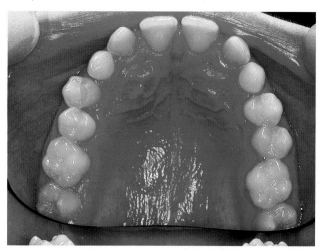

Fig. 5.2 (a) Lower occlusal view.

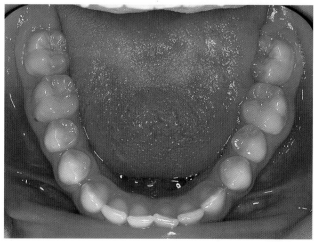

Fig. 5.2 (b) Upper occlusal view.

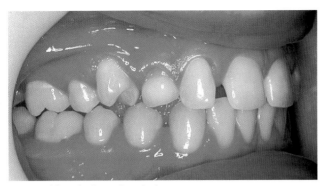

Fig. 5.2 (c) Right buccal occlusion.

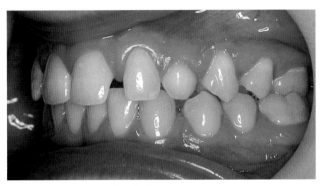

Fig. 5.2 (d) Left buccal occlusion.

Oral hygiene is fair with mild marginal gingival erythema related to $\underline{2|2}$ and the upper left buccal segment teeth.

No obvious buccal swellings in the $\underline{c}$ areas but there seems to be mucosal swellings palatal to $\underline{c2|c2}$, perhaps indicating the position of unerupted $\underline{3}$'s.

Slight enamel decalcification buccally on $\underline{6|6}$.

$$\frac{7\ 6\ 5\ 4\ c\ 2\ 1\ |\ 1\ 2\ c\ 4\ 5\ 6\ 7}{7\ 6\ 5\ 4\ 3\ 2\ 1\ |\ 1\ 2\ 3\ 4\ 5\ 6\ 7}\ \text{erupted.}$$

Mild lower labial segment crowding; $\overline{1|1}$ mesiolabially rotated; lower buccal segments spaced.

Upper arch uncrowded; spacing in the upper labial segment.

Class I incisor relationship with a centreline shift (clinically the lower centreline was 1 mm to the left).

Buccal segment relationship Class I bilaterally with $\overline{4|}$ in lingual crossbite with $\underline{4|}$; $\underline{|6}$ is in buccal crossbite with $\overline{|6}$.

What are the potential causes of $\underline{c}$'s being retained?

Absence of $\underline{3}$'s. This is highly unlikely (0.3% of Caucasians).

Ectopic position of $\underline{3}$'s—this is the most likely cause (1–2% in Caucasians with 8% of these bilateral).

What factors are implicated in maxillary canine ectopia?

The aetiology of maxillary canine ectopia is obscure but most probably multifactorial. Possible causatic factors are:

1. Genetic—palatally displaced $\underline{3}$ appears to result from a polygenic multifactorial mode of inheritance, with associated anomalies including incisor–premolar hypodontia and peg-shaped $\underline{2}$ (see below). Class II division 2 malocclusion is also associated with an increased incidence of palatal $\underline{3}$.
2. Crypt displacement—where the position of $\underline{3}$ is grossly displaced, this may be an aetiological factor.
3. $\underline{3}$ has the longest path of eruption of any permanent tooth.
4. Arch length discrepancy—palatal displacement of $\underline{3}$'s has been mostly associated with an uncrowded or spaced arch. Note the spacing present in Diane's upper arch.
5. Trauma to the maxillary anterior area at an early stage of development—this has been suggested but there is no history of trauma in this case.
6. Peg-shaped, short-rooted $\underline{2}$'s or absent $\underline{2}$'s – guidance for $\underline{3}$ is reduced where these features are evident, doubling the incidence of palatal impaction of $\underline{3}$.

Key point

● Palatal displacement of $\underline{3}$ is more common in an uncrowded arch and is associated with small, absent or abnormal root formation of $\underline{2}$'s and Class II division 2 malocclusion.

Note in Diane's case, the mesiodistal width of $\underline{2}$'s were the same as those of $\overline{2}$'s, indicating that $\underline{2}$'s are smaller than average and that a tooth-size discrepancy exists between upper and lower labial segment teeth.

Investigations
What investigations would you undertake regarding the retained $\underline{c}$'s? Explain why

It would be essential to determine if $\underline{3}$'s are present and to localize their position. Initial assessment should be clinical, and where suspicion of $\underline{3}$ displacement exists, radiographic examination should follow.

● Clinical

Palpation of the buccal sulci and palatal mucosae in the upper canine regions, as well as observation of the $\underline{2}$ inclination, usually provides a reasonable guide to the probable position of an unerupted $\underline{3}$. Labial displacement of $\underline{2}$ crown indicates $\underline{3}$ to be lying high and buccal over $\underline{2}$ root or low and palatal.

● Radiographic

Two films taken with either a vertical or a horizontal tube shift are required to assess accurately the location of unerupted 3's. A dental panoramic tomogram (DPT) gives a general good assessment of 3 position, although its potential for alignment is presented more favourably. The root length of c, vertical and mesiodistal position of 3 relative to the incisor roots, the axial inclination and apex location should be assessed. An anterior maxillary occlusal radiograph or a periapical film of each 3 is useful for detecting incisor resorption and determining the prognosis of the c's. Either of these views, used in combination with the panoramic view and application of parallax (a palatal 3 moves with the tube shift), can be used to locate 3's.

A lateral cephalometric radiograph is not indicated in Diane's case, but where it is justified on clinical grounds it provides valuable information about the position of 3's when used in combination with the panoramic view.

Diane's DPT and standard occlusal radiographs are shown in Figure 5.3. What are the features of note?

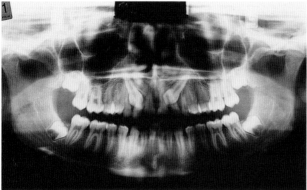

Fig. 5.3 (a) Dental panoramic tomogram.

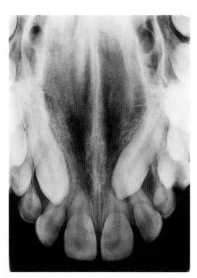

Fig. 5.3 (b) Standard occlusal radiograph.

Four developing third molars.
Presence of 3|3 , which are palatal.
Resorption of the roots of c|c .

Is there any way in which ectopia of 3's may be intercepted?

Early detection of an abnormal eruption path of 3 is essential in order to provide, if appropriate, an opportunity for interceptive measures to be undertaken. From 9 years, palpation for unerupted 3's should be carried out routinely. Importantly, the position of 3 must be localized before considering any interceptive extractions. Radiographic investigation is required when a difference is detected on clinical palpation of the upper buccal sulcus between opposite sides of the arch.

Where 3 is displaced palatally in an uncrowded arch, in a child aged 10–13 years old, removal of c may lead to 3 reverting to a normal path of eruption. The amount of improvement depends on the degree of overlap of 3 over 2 root, with a better prognosis when 3 overlies the distal rather than the mesial half of 2 root. Although improvement in 3 position may occur even where 3 is markedly displaced, specialist advice must be obtained before removal of c. Consideration must be given to balancing the extraction of c with removal of the opposite c to prevent a centreline shift. Normally, following extraction of c, clinical and radiographic re-evaluation should be undertaken at 6-monthly intervals. If no improvement in 3 position is observed on a DPT within 12 months, alternative treatment is required.

> **Key point**
>
> ● Removal of c's between 10 and 13 years may encourage improvement in the position of a palatally ectopic canine.

When 3 displacement is associated with crowding, elimination of crowding and space maintenance, if required, may stimulate 3 position to improve.

> **Key point**
>
> In planning treatment for a palatally ectopic canine, assess the following on radiograph:
> ● The root length of c.
> ● The vertical and mesiodistal position relative to the incisor roots.
> ● The axial inclination.
> ● The apex location.

Treatment
What management options are there for Diane's unerupted 3's? What are the indications for each option?

These are summarized in **Table 5.1**.

Table 5.1 Management options, with indications, for palatally displaced unerupted 3̲'s

Option	Indications	Comments
Early removal of c̲'s	See comments above in relation to interceptive treatment	Not a viable option in this case as Diane is 15 years old
Retain 3̲ and observe	Patient not keen for treatment Pathology or resorption of adjacent teeth not evident Good aesthetics/prognosis of c̲'s or 2̲ and 4̲ in good contact 3̲ severely displaced with no associated pathology evident	Need to monitor radiographically the unerupted 3̲ for cystic degeneration and/or root resorption of incisors
Surgical exposure of 3̲'s and orthodontic alignment	Highly motivated patient with excellent general dental health Spaced arch or possible to create space; vertical, anteroposterior and transverse position of 3̲ crown and root favourable	Prognosis is good: the nearer 3̲ is to the occlusal plane, 3̲ overlaps at most the distal half of 1̲ root, when 3̲ long axis is ≥ 30° to the midsagittal plane, when root of 3̲ is not dilacerated or ankylosed or 3̲ apex is not more distal than 5̲. Bond gold chain, bracket or magnet to 3̲ at surgery; alignment of 3̲ may commence with removable appliance but fixed appliance usually required to align 3̲ apex.
Remove 3̲	Patient not keen for alignment of 3̲ and radiographic evidence of associated cystic degeneration Hopeless prognosis for alignment of 3̲ 2̲ and 4̲ in good contact, or good root length on c̲ with good aesthetics or patient willing to undergo fixed appliance therapy to substitute 4̲ for 3̲ Early resorption of adjacent teeth	Prosthetic replacement of c̲ required when lost
Transplant 3̲	Adequate space in arch for 3̲ Intact removal of 3̲ possible Adequate buccal/palatal bone	Prognosis best if root of 3̲ is 50–75% formed, minimal handling of 3̲ root at surgery, and rigid splinting is avoided

Key point

- Surgical exposure and orthodontic alignment of a palatal 3̲ requires a well-disposed patient with good oral hygiene and dentition.

Which option would you favour?

As Diane is a highly motivated patient with a high standard of general dental care and the roots of c̲'s are resorbing with 3̲'s in reasonably favourable positions for orthodontic alignment, surgical exposure of 3̲'s and orthodontic alignment would be optimal.

What are the ideal aims of treatment?

Alignment of 3̲'s .
Build up 2̲'s to increase mesiodistal width.
Correction of crossbite of 4̲|6̲ .
Correction of lower centreline shift.

For treatment planning, Diane should be seen by an orthodontist, oral surgeon and restorative colleague to discuss management of 3̲'s and 2̲'s. Orthodontic alignment of 3̲'s, following their surgical exposure, was agreed. Build up of 2̲'s mesially was to precede this. Mid-treatment, after 3̲'s were across the occlusion, build-up of 2̲'s distally was planned.

The need for lower centreline correction should be reassessed following crossbite correction on $\frac{4}{4}|$.

How would you proceed with treatment?

Create space for 3̲'s alignment. This will be obtained by moving 2̲|2̲ slightly mesially. As they are distally inclined, mesial tipping only is required. These movements as well as palatal movement of 4̲| and buccal movement of |6̲ , could be accomplished easily by upper removable appliance therapy.

Detail the design of a suitable removable appliance
Activation

Palatal finger springs (0.5 mm stainless steel wire to move 2̲'s mesially).
Buccally approaching spring (0.7 mm stainless steel wire) with 'u' loop to 4̲| .
Screw section to move |6̲ buccally.

Retention

Adams clasps 6̲|6̲ (0.7 mm stainless steel wire).
Southend clasp 1̲|1̲ (0.7 mm stainless steel wire).

Anchorage

From baseplate.

Baseplate

Full palatal acrylic coverage

Posterior bite platforms ~2 mm in thickness to facilitate crossbite correction on 4|6. The acrylic needs to be relieved palatal and occlusal to 4|.

What instructions would you give the patient regarding turning of the screw?

It should be turned one quarter turn once per week (this is ~0.25 mm)

When the crossbites on 4|6 have been corrected what would you do?

Reduce the posterior capping to half its height at one visit and then remove it completely at the following visit to allow the posterior occlusion to settle. It would then be advisable to place an upper fixed appliance. A transpalatal arch, attached to bands on 6's, should be cemented for anchorage. Brackets should be bonded to all other upper teeth except 7 c|c 7 and alignment continued until a rectangular stainless steel stabilizing archwire (019 × 025 stainless steel in an 022 slot) can be placed.

Then arrange for surgical exposure of 3's.

What methods of surgical exposure are there?

Three methods exist:

1. Open surgical exposure followed by spontaneous eruption. 3 needs to be of correct inclination for this to succeed.
2. Open surgical exposure of 3 with packing. About 1 week postoperatively the pack is removed and an attachment is bonded to 3 to facilitate alignment with a fixed appliance.
3. Closed surgical exposure of 3 with attachment bonded during surgery. An eyelet or gold chain bonded to the mid-buccal aspect of 3 crown has the best prospect of bond survival.

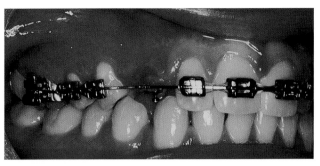

Fig. 5.4 Mid-treatment.

How may the 3's be aligned?

Elastic traction may be applied from the attachment bonded to 3's to the archwire (**Fig. 5.4**). Light forces (20–60 g) should be used. When movement of 3's is evident, c's should be extracted. Once 3's are close to the line of the arch, a bracket should be bonded to the mid-buccal aspect of each tooth. It is essential that the roots of 3's are adequately torqued to finalize their positioning.

What factors may you consider for retaining 3's in their corrected positions?

Aside from full correction of torque, early correction of rotations should be undertaken followed by circumferential fiberotomy to 3's and then the provision of a bonded retainer.

Recommended reading

Ericson S, Kurol J 1988 Early treatment of palatally erupting maxillary canines by extraction of the primary canines. Eur J Orthod 10:283–295.

Kokich VG, Spear FM 1997 Guidelines for managing the orthodontic – restorative patient. Semin Orthod 3:3–20.

McSherry PF 1998 The ectopic maxillary canine: a review. Br J Orthod 25:209–216.

For revision see Mind Map 5, page 151

6

Infra-occluded primary molars

Summary

Aileen is 11. She is referred by her general dental practitioner regarding infra-occluded lower primary molars (**Fig. 6.1**). What is the cause and how would you treat it?

History

● Complaint

Aileen is unconcerned by the position of her back teeth.

● History of complaint

Aileen and her mother were unaware of any problem with the molar teeth until this was brought to their attention recently by their general dental practitioner. There is no discomfort associated with these teeth and they are not loose.

● Medical history

Aileen is fit and well.

● Dental history

She is a regular attender at the family's general dental practitioner. No dental treatment has been required to date.

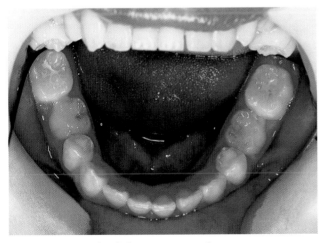

Fig. 6.1 Lower occlusal view at presentation.

● Family history

Aileen's mother has several permanent teeth missing and these have been replaced by bridgework.

Examination

● Extraoral examination

Aileen has a mild Class II skeletal pattern with average FMPA and no facial asymmetry. The lips are incompetent with the lower lip lying at the incisal edges of the upper incisors. There are no temporomandibular joint signs or symptoms.

● Intraoral examination

Soft tissues of the tongue, floor of mouth, palate/oropharynx and the oral mucosa are healthy. The intraoral views are shown in **Figures 6.1** and **6.2**.

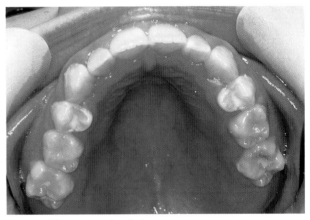

Fig. 6.2 (a) Upper occlusal view.

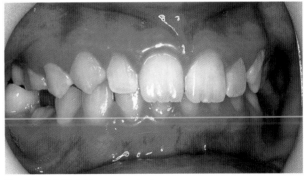

Fig. 6.2 (b) Right buccal occlusion.

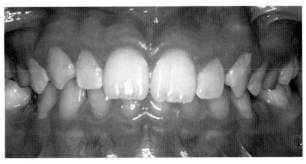

Fig. 6.2 (c) Anterior occlusion.

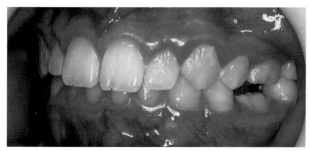

Fig. 6.2 (d) Left buccal occlusion.

What do you see?

Plaque deposits on many teeth with associated marginal gingival erythema.

Dentition appears caries-free; fissure sealants are present occlusally in the first permanent molars.

Uncrowded lower labial segment; e|e infra-occluded; uncrowded upper arch; e|e present.

Mild Class II division 1 incisor relationship (overjet is 45 mm measured clinically); overbite slightly increased and complete.

Lower centreline to the right.

First molar relationship: right half unit Class II with 6e| in crossbite; left Class I.

What is the prevalence of infra-occlusion of primary molars?

It is between 8% and 14%.

Why does infra-occlusion of primary molars occur?

Separate phases of resorption and repair occur in the exfoliation of primary teeth. Although resorption predominates in most cases, sometimes repair prevails temporarily leading to ankylosis of a primary molar. As alveolar growth and eruption of the adjacent teeth continue, the tooth infra-occludes.

Key point

Infra-occlusion of a primary molar is due to:
● Ankylosis of the tooth while alveolar growth and eruption of the adjacent teeth continues.

Investigations
What investigations would you undertake? Explain why
● **Clinical**

Assess:
1. Mobility of e's—if these are mobile this tends to indicate that they are close to exfoliation and that the permanent successors are present.
2. Extent of infra-occlusion of e's—if these teeth are in danger of submerging below gingival level, their

removal is indicated. (For grading of infra-occlusion, see page 92.)
3. If e's ankylosed. Typically a 'tin-can' sound is audible when the occlusal surface is percussed with the handle end of a dental mirror and the sound compared to that obtained from percussion of adjacent fully erupted teeth.
4. Overeruption of opposing teeth—this could lead to interferences in functional occlusion and present difficulties if prosthetic replacement of e's spaces is required in the absence of 5's.

Key point

With submerged e's, assess:
● Mobility of e's.
● Extent of infra-occlusion.
● If e's are ankylosed.
● Overeruption of opposing teeth.
● If 5's are present.

● **Radiographic**

1. A dental panoramic tomogram—to determine if unerupted teeth are present, in normal developmental position and of normal form and size.
2. A lateral cephalometric radiograph may be required later if fixed appliance therapy is planned and the patient is keen to proceed. It would allow more accurate determination of the skeletal pattern in the anteroposterior and vertical dimensions and for the incisor angulations to be assessed.

Both e's were found to be non-mobile and were not infra-occluded below gingival level, but clinically both were ankylosed.

The dental panoramic tomogram is shown in Figure 6.3. What are the findings of note?

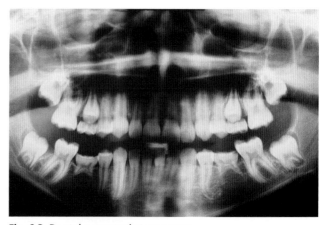

Fig. 6.3 Dental panoramic tomogram.

- Dental development corresponds with chronological age.
- Extensive resorption of the roots of e's; short roots on e̅'s.
- Absent 5̅'s and all third molars.
- Absence of periodontal ligament space related to e̅|e̅ .

Which teeth does hypodontia affect most commonly?

The prevalence of hypodontia in the permanent dentition is 3.5–6.5%. The most distal tooth of any tooth type is usually affected, i.e. the lateral incisor, the second premolar, the third molar. In Caucasians, third molars are most commonly affected (25–35%) followed by 5̅ (3%) and then 2̲ (2%). Females are affected more than males and tooth size in the remainder of the dentition tends to be reduced.

Key point

Hypodontia:
- Prevalence: 3.5–6.5% in permanent dentition.
- Frequency: 8's, then 5̅, 2̲.
- Females more than males.

Following perusal of the panoramic tomogram and preliminary discussion of treatment options with Aileen and her mother, a lateral cephalometric radiograph was taken. Analysis revealed the following:

SNA = 82°; SNB = 76.5°; ANB° = 5.5°; 1̲ to maxillary plane = 112°; 1̅ to mandibular plane = 92°; MMPA = 26°; Facial % = 55%.

What do these values tell you? (see p. 185)

They confirm the clinical impression of a mild Class II skeletal pattern with average FMPA. Incisor inclinations to their underlying dental bases are also within the normal range.

Diagnosis
What is your diagnosis?

Class II division I malocclusion on a mild Class II skeletal base with average FMPA. Generalized marginal gingivitis, uncrowded lower arch with submerged e̅'s. Uncrowded upper arch. First molar relationship right half unit Class II with 6e̲| in crossbite; left Class I. Hypodontia of 5̅'s and third molars.

What is the IOTN DHC grade (see p. 183)?

4h due to absent 5̅'s.

Treatment
What treatment options are there for the lower arch? Explain why

In view of the lack of crowding:
1. Accept the position and status of e̅|e̅ , realizing their poor long-term prognosis due to the short root length, but build up e̅|e̅ with occlusal inlays to bring them into occlusion. This procedure has been shown to improve longevity of infra-occluded molars. When eventually they are lost, resin-retained or conventional bridgework or implants can be used to replace the missing units. The girl and her mother would need to be aware of the implications of this treatment proposal over the lifetime of the dentition including the need for replacement of any prosthesis as required.
2. Extract e̅|e̅ in view of their poor long-term prognosis and as infra-occlusion is likely to progress with absence of 5̅'s. Then, close the extraction spaces with a lower fixed appliance. This has the advantage of removing the need for a prosthesis but a retainer would need to be worn post-treatment for several years at night to minimize the likelihood of space opening. Alternatively bonded retainers could be placed on the buccal aspects of 6 4̲|4 6 to maintain space closure.

What implications do these options have for the upper arch?

If e̅'s are retained, the slight overjet increase could be accepted as the teeth are aligned and provided the patient is in agreement.

If e̅'s are to be extracted and a lower fixed appliance planned, it would be sensible to resort to an upper premolar extraction on either side in the upper arch (probably 5̲'s in view of the small overjet and absence of crowding, although it will be necessary to await their eruption) and proceed to fixed appliance therapy to achieve Class I molar and incisor relationships.

Following discussion, Aileen and her mother decided to proceed with fixed appliance therapy (**Fig. 6.4**) after Aileen's oral hygiene improved following several visits to the hygenist.

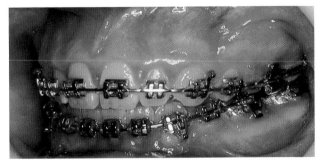

Fig. 6.4 Fixed appliances.

The occlusion following removal of e|e , then 5|5 and e̅'s and fixed appliance therapy is shown in **Figure 6.5**.

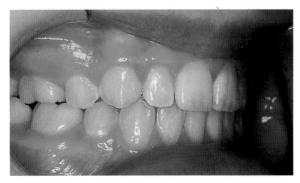

Fig. 6.5 a

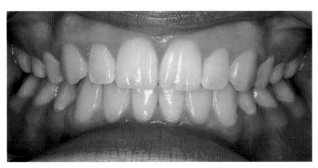

Fig. 6.5 b

Fig. 6.5 c

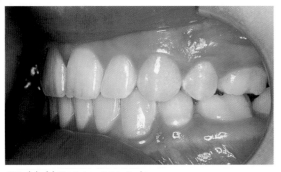

Fig. 6.5 (a)–(c) Post-treatment views.

If 5̅'s had been present radiographically, what would have been your treatment plan?

Ankylosis of e̅'s is likely to be temporary when permanent successors exist, and e̅'s should exfoliate within a normal time frame. The position of e̅'s should be monitored until then, and if the infra-occlusion progresses extraction is recommended, particularly if the crown of e̅ moves to lie below gingival level (reinclusion)and/or apical closure is almost complete on 5̅.

Key point

Management options for infra-occluded e̅:
- 5̅ present, no reinclusion: allow e̅ to exfoliate.
- 5̅ present, and reinclusion: extract or surgically remove e̅.
- 5̅ absent: retain and place onlay
    extract and space close.
    extract and prosthetic replacement.

Recommended reading

Bjerklin K, Bennett J 2000 The long-term survival of lower second primary molars in subjects with agenesis of the premolars. Eur J Orthod 22:245–255.

Kurol J, Koch K 1986 The effect of extraction of infraoccluded deciduous molars: a longitudinal study. Am J Orthod 87:46–55.

For revision see Mind Map 6, page 152

7

Increased overjet

Summary

Emma, aged 11, is teased at school about her prominent upper front teeth (**Fig. 7.1**). What are the possible causes and how may it be treated?

History

● Complaint

Emma's upper front teeth stick out. Her mother is very concerned about her daughter's appearance and is anxious for her to be treated.

● History of complaint

The upper front teeth have always been prominent, even when the primary incisors were present. Emma is teased about her teeth at school and the teasing is upsetting her. She recently fell in the school yard and hit her two upper front teeth on the ground. Fortunately there was only minimal incisal enamel damage to 1|1.

Medical history

Emma has suffered from asthma since she was 4 years old. This is managed by taking Ventolin.

Key point

- Increased overjet may predispose to teasing and upper incisor trauma.

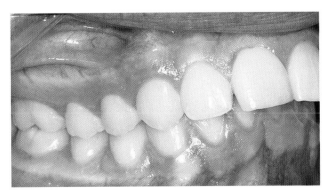

Fig. 7.1 Right buccal occlusion at presentation.

Examination

● Extraoral

Emma's full-face and profile views are shown in **Figure 7.2**.

How would you assess Emma's skeletal pattern?

The skeletal pattern is the relationship of the mandibular to the maxillary dental base in all three planes of space—anteroposterior, vertical and lateral. With the patient seated upright with the Frankfort plane (superior aspect of the external auditory meatus to the inferior aspect of the orbital margin) horizontal, the lips in repose and the teeth in maximum interdigitation, assessment should be as follows:

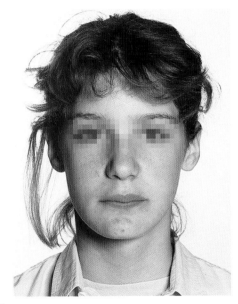

Fig. 7.2 a

Fig. 7.2 b

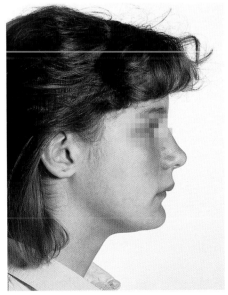

Fig. 7.2 (a) Full-face. (b) Profile.

1. *Anteroposterior*. Viewing the soft tissue facial profile in most cases allows the following classification to be made:
   Class I: the mandible lies 2–3 mm behind the maxilla.
   Class II: the mandible lies more than 2–3 mm behind the maxilla.
   Class III: the mandible lies less than 2–3 mm behind the maxilla.

Due to variation in lip thickness, this method is not always reliable and palpation of the alveolar bases over the apices of the upper and lower incisors in the midline has been claimed to give a better estimate of skeletal pattern.

Emma has a Class II skeletal pattern.

2. *Vertical*:
   Lower facial height. The distance from the mid eyebrow level to the base of the nose (upper face height) should equal that from the base of the nose to the inferior aspect of the chin (lower face height). The lower face height is reduced when the latter measurement is reduced and the converse is true when this distance is increased.
   Frankfort–mandibular planes angle (FMPA). With a finger along the inferior aspect of the mandible and a ruler placed along the Frankfort plane, project both of these lines backwards in the imagination to estimate the FMPA. The FMPA is then classified as average (both lines intersect at the back of the skull, occiput), reduced (both lines meet beyond occiput) or increased (both lines meet anterior to occiput).

Emma has a slightly reduced lower facial height and FMPA.

3. *Transverse*. Stand directly behind the patient and look down across the face, checking the coincidence of the midlines of the nose, upper and lower lips and midpoint of the chin. Alternatively assess the face from in front. It is important to note that slight facial asymmetry is common. The location (upper, middle or lower facial third) and extent of any asymmetry should be recorded: There is no facial asymmetry.

No mandibular deviation on closure or temporomandibular signs/symptoms were detected.

The lips are habitually competent with the lower lip tending to lie under the upper incisors at rest (Fig. 7.2b).

● **Intraoral**

The intraoral views are shown in Figures 7.1 *and 7.3. What do these show?*

There are plaque deposits on several teeth and overall mild marginal gingival erythema.

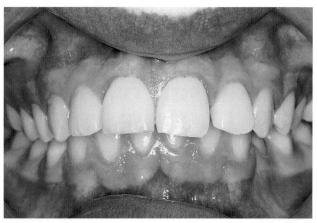

Fig. 7.3 a

Fig. 7.3 b

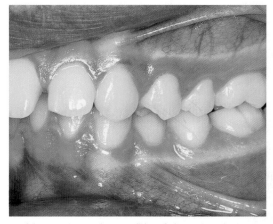

Fig. 7.3 (a) Anterior occlusion. (b) Left buccal occlusion.

All teeth appear to be good quality.
She is in the permanent dentition with
$$\frac{6\,5\,4\,3\,2\,1\,|\,1\,2\,3\,4\,5\,6}{6\,5\,4\,3\,2\,1\,|\,1\,2\,3\,4\,5\,6}$$ present. $\overline{7|7}$ are erupting.
The upper and lower arches are uncrowded.
There is a Class II division I incisor relationship with increased overjet (measured 7 mm clinically); the overbite is increased and complete. The buccal segment relationship is a half unit Class II bilaterally. There is

a lingual crossbite (scissors bite) affecting $\dfrac{4}{4}$.

What are the causes of an increased overjet?

These are given in **Table 7.1**.

Investigation
What radiographs are indicated?

A panoramic radiograph is required to check the presence, position, developmental stage and abnormalities of crown and root of any unerupted teeth. Untreated caries should also be noted and bitewing radiographs requested, if necessary. In view of the history of trauma to the upper incisor area, a periapical view or an upper anterior occlusal radiograph should be taken and examined for possible apical pathology.

Table 7.1 Causes of an increased overjet

Cause	Aetiology
Skeletal pattern	May be Class I, II or III
	If Class II, mandibular deficiency is almost entirely the primary cause but may be excessive horizontal maxillary growth or a combination of the two factors
Soft tissues[a]	Lower lip lying under the upper incisors to create an anterior oral seal will procline the upper incisors and retrocline the lower incisors (likely if there is a Class II skeletal pattern, reduced lower facial height and lip incompetence)
	Hyperactive lower lip will retrocline the lower incisors
	Primary atypical swallowing pattern (endogenous tongue thrust) will tend to procline upper (but also lower) incisors
Digit sucking habit	If present for more than 6 hours out of 24, it will procline upper incisors, retrocline lower incisors, create an anterior open bite and a tendency to buccal segment crossbite
	Overjet increase is often asymmetric due to digit positioning
Crowding	Labial displacement of upper incisors and/or lingual displacement of lower incisors
Any combination of above	

[a] Effects determined principally by the skeletal pattern, and thereafter by the manner in which an anterior oral seal is produced.

A lateral cephalometric radiograph is indicated as there is an anteroposterior and a vertical skeletal discrepancy. In addition, anteroposterior movement of the incisors is planned.

The findings of the cephalometric analysis are:

$SNA = 82°$; $SNB = 76°$; SN to max. plane $= 9°$; MMPA $= 22°$; $\underline{1}$ to max. plane $= 114°$; $\overline{1}$ to mand. plane $= 92°$; Facial % $= 52\%$.

What do these indicate?

ANB value of 6° (SNA minus SNB) indicates a Class II skeletal pattern.

Reduced MMPA and Facial % (normal value is 55° + 2°).

Upper incisors of above average inclination and slightly retroclined lower incisors. Although within the normal range the $\overline{1}$ to mand. plane must be considered with the MMPA as there is an inverse relationship between the two values. $\overline{1}$ to mand. plane (93°) and MMPA (27°) should total 120° or

alternatively $\overline{1}$ to mand. plane angle should be 120° – MMPA. Hence in this case, the $\overline{1}$ to mand. plane angle should be $120° - 22° = 98°$. At 92°, it is retroclined.

Would you consider any other investigations?

It would be wise to do sensibility tests of $1 | 1$. These proved positive for all tests, with no marked difference in recordings between teeth.

Diagnosis
What is the diagnosis?

Emma has a Class II division 1 malocclusion on a mild Class II skeletal base with reduced FMPA. Generalized marginal gingivitis. $1 | 1$ have suffered recent trauma. There is no crowding of the upper and lower arches. The buccal segment relationship is a half unit Class II bilaterally with a lingual crossbite of $\overline{|4}$.

What is the IOTN DHC score (see p. 183)?

4a due to overjet > 6 mm but ≤ 9 mm.

What factors predispose to upper incisor trauma?

The overjet increase—the risk is doubled where the overjet exceeds 9 mm.

Lip incompetence—this places the incisors at greater risk of trauma.

Sex of the patient—boys experience more upper incisor trauma than girls.

What are the aims of treatment?

To reduce the overbite and overjet to establish a Class I incisor relationship.

To correct the buccal segment relationship to Class I.

To correct the crossbite on $\dfrac{4}{|4}$.

What treatment would you advise? Explain why

Emma's malocclusion should be amenable to correction by growth modification with functional appliance therapy. Favourable features are the patient is likely to be growing and is approaching the pubertal growth spurt. The skeletal pattern is mildly Class II, due to mandibular retrusion rather than maxillary protrusion. The arches are uncrowded and aligned; the lower incisors are slightly retroclined; the buccal segment relationship is a half-unit Class II so a modest shift of the arch relationship is required for it to be corrected to Class I.

Functional appliances are usually contraindicated where the lower incisors are proclined, as they induce further proclination through generation of Class II intermaxillary traction. Following functional appliance therapy, fixed appliances may be required to detail the

Key point

A functional appliance:
● Aims to 'modify' growth.
● Is only effective in growing children, preferably just pre-pubertal.

occlusion. It would be advisable then to retain the result by night-only wear of a functional appliance until growth is complete.

Describe the records you would take to allow fabrication of the functional appliance?

The records required are upper and lower impressions as well as a wax registration taken with the mandible postured forward about 4–6 mm, the bite open about 2–3 mm and with no appreciable shift in the upper and lower dental midlines. This 'working bite' may be recorded by softening several layers of wax in hot water, forming this to a horseshoe shape indexed firmly over the upper teeth and finally guiding the mandible to the correct anteroposterior and vertical position by checking the relationship of the centrelines and the incisal opening. Alternatively, layers of wax may be adapted to a proprietary bite registration fork, which has graduated markings to facilitate assessment of the postured mandibular position. The wax registration should then be chilled, examined for adequate dental registration and re-checked for accuracy in the mouth before forwarding with the impressions to the laboratory.

On issuing the functional appliance, what instructions would you give Emma?

Assuming that this is a Twin-Block appliance, as this is now the most universally adopted type of functional appliance, the instructions would be as follows:

The appliance should be worn full-time, including at mealtimes, from insertion. The only time it is removed is after meals for cleaning and also for contact sports, during which time it should be stored in a hard plastic tub.

Speaking and eating will be difficult for the first few days but will improve if you persevere.

You must avoid eating hard or sticky foods or consuming fizzy drinks while wearing the appliance as these are likely to damage the appliance and/or your teeth. The appliance and the teeth should be cleaned thoroughly after every meal.

Mild jaw discomfort and muscle tenderness are common for the first few days but reduce after that. It may be necessary to take a mild analgesic, as required, during this 'settling-in' period.

Should a sore spot develop or there be any breakage of the appliance, you should return immediately to have any adjustments carried out.

How does a Twin-Block work and what effects does it produce?

The Twin-Block appliance consists of upper and lower appliances incorporating buccal blocks with interfacing inclined planes (at about 70°), which posture the mandible forward on closure (**Fig. 7.4**). This appliance works by using the forces generated by the orofacial musculature, tooth eruption and dentofacial growth. The upper midline expansion screw is usually adjusted once per week by the patient until the arch widths are coordinated with the mandible postured forward in a Class I incisor relationship. In this case no expansion was required in view of the scissors bite on $\frac{4}{4}$. The effects are usually as follows:

● **Skeletal**

Forward growth of the mandible.
Lower anterior facial height increase.

● **Dental**

Retroclination of upper incisors/proclination of lower incisors.
Promotion of mesial and upward eruption of lower posterior teeth (see below).
Distal movement of the upper molars.
Upper arch expansion.

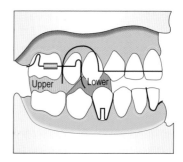

(a)

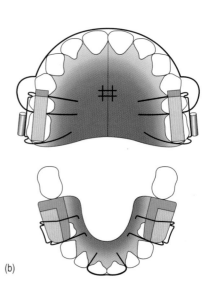

(b)

Fig. 7.4 Design of a Twin-Block appliance.

Key point

A functional appliance for Class II correction:
● Postures the mandible downward and forward.
● Generates intermaxillary traction.
● Uses, removes or modifies forces of the orofacial musculature, tooth eruption and dentofacial growth.

Following overjet correction by Twin-Block therapy, what occlusal anomaly is usually manifest posteriorly in the dental arches?

A posterior open bite is usually present bilaterally due to the buccal blocks.

How may this be corrected?

There are three possible means available to allow correction of the posterior open bite by eruption of the buccal segment teeth:

The patient may be instructed to proceed to part-time wear of the appliance.

The buccal blocks may be trimmed progressively over a period of a few months until a posterior occlusion is established.

Wear of the Twin-Blocks can be ceased and the patient fitted with an upper Hawley Retainer (Adams clasps 0.7 mm on 6|6 , labial bow 0.7 mm 3| to |3) with a steep anterior inclined biteplane, which aims to maintain overjet correction by posturing the mandible forward while encouraging eruption of the lower buccal segment teeth. Full-time wear of the appliance is required, except for contact sports and tooth cleaning, until a well-interdigitating posterior occlusion is established. Then night-only wear of the appliance, until growth has ceased or until a second phase of treatment commences, is permissible.

If there is no progress at 6 months, what action would you take?

Lack of overjet correction could be due to poor patient response to the appliance, improper design or poor compliance. Treatment should be discontinued and a re-evaluation made. The patient's standing height should be recorded and compared to the pretreatment measurement. This will give an indication of growth over the intervening period. Provided Emma remains keen for orthodontic treatment, new records, including a progress cephalometric radiograph, should be taken and analysed to allow a new treatment plan to be devised.

What other treatment options are there?

If a *design problem* with the appliance is identified as the cause of lack of treatment progress, then remaking the appliance incorporating appropriate design modifications could be undertaken and treatment recommenced.

If *poor compliance* is to blame for no progress, then the reason(s) should be ascertained from discussion with the child. If lack of motivation or interest in treatment is the cause, it would be prudent to avoid any further appliance therapy until such time as the child has a change of heart regarding orthodontic treatment.

Orthodontic camouflage—by retraction of the upper incisors into first premolar extraction spaces, accepting the Class II skeletal pattern. Importantly, this treatment should not be detrimental to facial aesthetics. Although some amount of tipping movement of the upper incisors is permissible, fixed appliances would be required to ensure an optimal interincisal angle is created. A useful rule of thumb with tipping movement is that each millimetre of incisor retraction approximates to a 2.5° change in axial inclination. With an original overjet of 8 mm and a target overjet of 3 mm (representing a 5 mm reduction), this would equate to a 12.5° change producing a final incisor inclination of 101.5°. This value is outside the normal range (109° ± 6°) and the incisors would be quite upright. An upper incisor angulation of 95° to the maxillary plane is regarded as the limit for acceptable retraction by tipping movements.

What factors govern stability of the corrected overjet?

For the best prospects of stability the interincisal angle should be within normal limits (135° ± 10°) and the overjet completely reduced with the incisors in soft tissue balance, i.e. no tongue thrust and the lower lip covering at least one third of the labial surface of the upper incisors. A period of retention will nonetheless be required and this should extend until growth is complete following functional appliance therapy.

Key point

After functional appliance therapy:
● Ensure the upper incisors are in soft tissue balance and controlled by the lower lip.
● Retain until growth is complete.

The profile and occlusion following functional appliance therapy are shown in **Figure 7.5**.

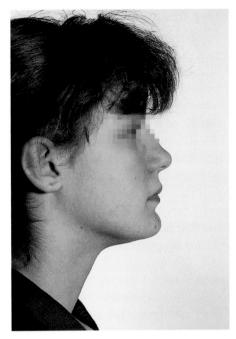

Fig. 7.5 a

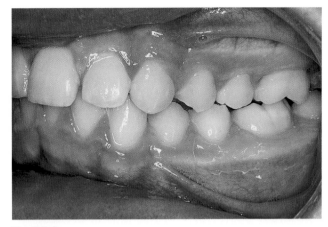

Fig. 7.5 b

Fig. 7.5 c

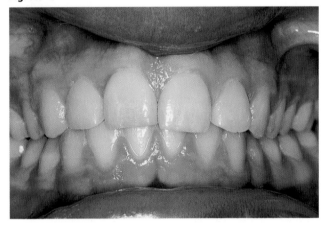

Fig. 7.5 After functional appliance therapy. (a) Profile. (b,c) Occlusion.

Recommended reading

Di Biase AT, Sandler PJ 2001 Malocclusion, orthodontics and bullying. Dent Update 28:464–466.

King GJ, Keeling SD, Hocevar RA, Wheeler TT 1990 The timing of treatment for Class II malocclusions in children: a literature review. Angle Orthod 60:87–97.

O'Brien KD et al 2003 Effectiveness of early orthodontic treatment with the Twin-block appliance: a multicentre, randomized controlled trial. Part 1: Dental and skeletal effects. Am J Orthod Dentofacial Orthop 124:234–243.

Tulloch JFC, Phillips C, Proffit WR 1998 Benefit of early Class II treatment. Progress report of a two-phase randomized clinical trial. Am J Orthod Dentofacial Orthop 113:62–72.

For revision see Mind Map 7, page 153

8

Incisor crossbite

Summary

Matthew is 8 years old. He presents with an upper incisor in crossbite (**Fig. 8.1**). What is the cause and how would you manage it?

History

● Complaint

Matthew's mother is concerned that her son's upper front teeth are not straight and is anxious for treatment to be undertaken soon.

● History of complaint

1| erupted inside the lower teeth. There is no history of a fall or other trauma to the primary predecessor or to 1| . a| was lost over a year ago, a little later than |a .

● Medical history

Matthew is in good health.

● Dental history

d| was extracted uneventfully under local anaesthesia 8 months ago.

Examination

● Extraoral

The skeletal pattern is Class I with an average FMPA. There is no facial asymmetry. The lips are competent.

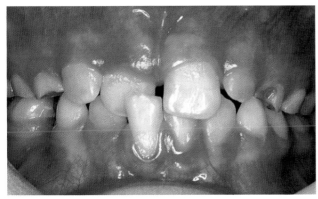

Fig. 8.1 Anterior occlusion at presentation.

There are no abnormal temporomandibular joint signs or symptoms.

● Intraoral

What features are visible on the intraoral views (Figs. 8.1, 8.2 a–c)?

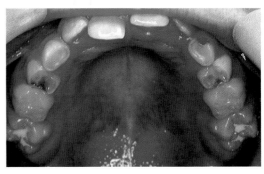

Fig. 8.2 a

Fig. 8.2 b

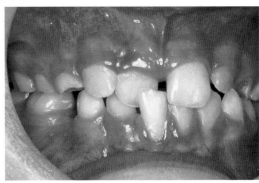

Fig. 8.2 c

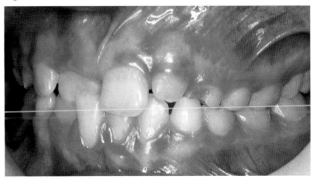

Fig. 8.2 (a) Upper occlusal view. (b) Right buccal occlusion. (c) Left buccal occlusion.

Oral hygiene is fair. The gingival appearance is consistent with mild marginal gingivitis related to the incisor teeth. d| has been lost. There is marked attrition of c|c with carious involvement of |c mesially and d|d distally.

Gingival recession appears to be evident on the labial aspect of 1| . 1| is displaced labially but otherwise the lower arch appears uncrowded. 2|2 are mesiolabially rotated; $\underline{1|}$ is displaced slightly palatally and there is a small median diastema. Otherwise the upper arch appears uncrowded. The incisor relationship is Class I and $\underline{1|}$ is in crossbite; $\underline{|2}$ is partially erupted with the disto-incisal aspect in crossbite with $\overline{|c}$.

What specific features would you check? Explain why

1. *The periodontal status of* $\overline{1|}$ —degree of mobility and pocket probing depth associated with $\overline{1|}$ should be assessed to determine its prognosis as it is being displaced labially by deflecting occlusal contact and gingival recession is present.

$\overline{1|}$ exhibited Grade 2 mobility but probing pocket depth was less than 2 mm indicating good periodontal prognosis in the event the crossbite relationship is corrected. For labial recession see p. 36.

2. *Can the patient achieve an edge-to-edge relationship on* $\dfrac{1|}{1}$? If so, this indicates that only a small amount of labial movement of $\underline{1|}$ is required to correct the crossbite relationship.

An edge-to-edge relationship of $\dfrac{1|}{1}$ was easily achievable by the patient.

3. *Is there a mandibular displacement on closure?* If the mandible is shifted anteriorly or laterally on closure from initial tooth contact, on $\dfrac{1|}{1}$ or $\dfrac{|2}{|c}$ respectively, into maximum interdigitation, early treatment to eliminate the displacement is indicated on dental health grounds. The rationale for this approach is that in susceptible individuals, mandibular displacement on closure due to premature tooth contact(s) may lead eventually to temporomandibular joint dysfunction syndrome.

A 3 mm anterior mandibular displacement on closure was detected from initial contact on $\dfrac{1|}{1}$; there was no lateral mandibular displacement associated with the crossbite affecting $\dfrac{|2}{|c}$.

4. *The amount of overbite on* $\underline{1|}$. As the amount of overbite post-treatment is a major factor governing stability of incisor crossbite correction and as overbite reduces when the incisor edge is moved upwards and forward during incisor proclination, a deep overbite pretreatment is a favourable feature. In this case the overbite was 3 mm on $\underline{1|}$ and there is a good prospect of adequate overbite following crossbite correction.

5. *The inclination of* $\underline{1|}$ —an upper incisor that is upright or retroclined is better for proclination than one that is already labially inclined. Further proclination of the latter may not be possible or could result in unfavourable occlusal loading.

6. *The amount of space required to procline* $\underline{1|}$ —space already exists in the upper incisor area and there is no need for any extractions.

Key point

Where an incisor crossbite is present, check:
- Periodontal status of lower incisors.
- If an edge-to-edge incisor occlusion is achievable.
- If mandibular displacement is present.
- Amount of overbite.
- Incisor inclination.
- Amount of space required for correction.

Investigations
What special investigations would you request? Why?

A dental panoramic tomogram would be required to check on the presence/absence of permanent teeth and whether there is a supernumerary tooth present in the upper midline. Should there be any suspicion of the latter, a maxillary anterior occlusal view should be taken to note the relation of the supernumerary tooth to the roots of the upper incisors. A periapical radiograph of the lower central incisors is not required as the clinical examination does not lend significant cause for concern to the prognosis of these teeth.

Bitewing radiographs should be taken to diagnose accurately the extent of carious involvement of the primary molars.

The dental panoramic tomogram taken by a previous general dental practitoner (6 months prior to this) is shown in Figure 8.3. What does it show?

Normal alveolar bone height except for apparent angular bone defects related to the mesial aspects

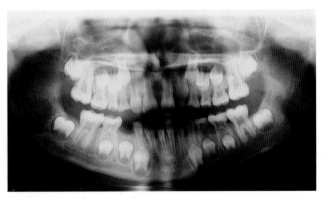

Fig. 8.3 Dental panoramic tomogram.

of $\overline{6|6}$. (Both teeth, however, were non-mobile and pocket depths were < 2 mm on the mesial and distal aspects of $\overline{6|6}$.)

$\overline{d|}$ absent; caries in $\frac{d|c\,d}{e|d\,e}$.

All permanent teeth (excep 8's) present, of normal size and in normal developmental positions.

Diagnosis
What is your diagnosis?

Matthew has a Class I malocclusion on a Class I dental base with average FMPA.

Mild marginal gingivitis related to the incisor teeth.

Gingival recession related to $\overline{1|}$ labially.

Caries in $\frac{d|c\,d}{e|d\,e}$.

Crossbite on $\underline{1|}$ with associated mandibular displacement.

Misalignment of upper and lower labial segments.

What is the IOTN DHC grade (see p. 183)?

4c due to mandibular displacement > 2 mm between the retruded contact position (RCP) and the intercuspal position (ICP).

What would you deem to be the prognosis for the labial recession related to $\overline{1|}$?

For accurate assessment of the extent of the labial recession, the soft tissues should be healthy, and at present gingival inflammation is evident. There appears, however, to be some attached gingiva labially and the recession does not extend to the sulcus reflection. It is also not associated with a frenal pull. At this stage, provided oral hygiene improves and the crossbite is corrected, the gingival recession should not worsen, although the width of attached gingiva will not increase.

Why is $\underline{1|}$ in crossbite?

This is most likely due to a slightly palatal ectopic position of $\underline{1|}$ tooth bud.

Treatment
What treatment would you provide and why?

1. *Oral hygiene instruction*—this is required to improve gingival health and to remove the plaque insult to the gingival recession related to $\overline{1|}$.
2. *Caries management*—a diet diary should be completed over three consecutive days (one of which should be a weekend day) and then appropriate dietary advice should be given based on the findings (see Chapter 19). Although several primary molars are carious, none have associated

symptoms. Restorative management of carious primary teeth is dealt with in Chapters 19 and 22.
3. Upper removable appliance therapy to procline $\underline{1|}$. Due to the mandibular displacement that is producing periodontal trauma to $\overline{1|}$, correction of the crossbite on $\underline{1|}$ is required urgently.
4. Monitor the lower centreline and consider removal of $\overline{|d}$ if a centreline shift develops.

Describe the appliance design you would use to align $\underline{1|}$

The appliance would have the following design:

Adams clasps $\underline{6d|d6}$ (clasps on $\underline{6|6}$ in 0.7 mm stainless steel wire; clasps on $\underline{d|d}$ in 0.6 mm wire).

Z spring (0.5 mm stainless steel wire) to procline $\underline{1|}$.

Acrylic baseplate with full palatal coverage incorporating posterior capping (~2 mm in height).

The appliance is shown in **Figure 8.4**.

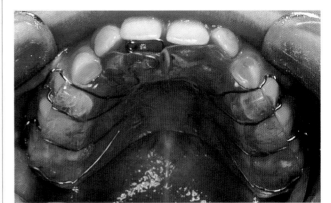

Fig. 8.4 Upper removable appliance to procline $\underline{1|}$.

What will determine stability of crossbite correction on $\underline{1|}$?

Provided there is 2–3 mm of overbite on $\underline{1|}$ following proclination, the prospect of stability is good. Subsequent mandibular growth must also be favourable.

The occlusion following crossbite correction on $\underline{1|}$ is shown in **Figure 8.5**.

Key point

Early treatment of an incisor crossbite is advisable if:
- There is associated mandibular displacement and/or periodontal trauma.

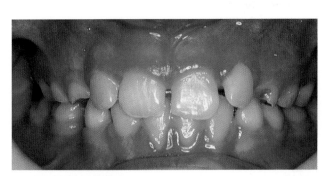

Fig. 8.5 Post-treatment.

Recommended reading

Gravely JF 1984 A study of the mandibular closure path in Angle Class III relationship. Br J Orthod 11:85–91.

For revision see Mind Map 8, page 154

9

Reverse overjet

Summary

Alistair, 8.5 years old, presents with a reverse overjet on all of his upper incisors (**Fig. 9.1**). What is the cause and how may it be treated?

History

● Complaint

Alistair is not bothered about the way his teeth bite together and is not concerned about any aspect of his facial appearance. His father, however, feels that Alistair's chin is somewhat prominent and gives the boy an aggressive-looking appearance. Sometimes Alistair is teased about his chin at school.

● History of complaint

Alistair's upper permanent incisors erupted behind his lower teeth. His mother's recollection is that the bite of his 'milk' teeth was similar. Alistair is not bothered by the occasional teasing he gets about his chin.

Alistair's parents are keen for treatment, if possible, at this stage to correct his bite and reduce the prominence of his chin, which would remove the source of teasing at school.

● Medical history

Alistair is fit and well.

● Family history

Alistair's father reports that his own teeth meet in a manner similar to the boy's and he also has a slightly prominent chin but is unconcerned by it. His father had orthodontic treatment with extraction of two lower teeth and fixed appliances when he was a teenager to correct the bite of his front teeth. His bite changed a lot after he stopped wearing the retainers.

Examination

● Extraoral

Alistair has a mild Class III skeletal pattern with average FMPA (**Fig. 9.2**) and no facial asymmetry.

What other features would you check for?

The presence/absence of a mandibular displacement on closure.
Alistair could just achieve an edge-to-edge incisor relationship.
Temporomandibular signs/symptoms.

A 3 mm anterior mandibular displacement on $\underline{1|1}$ was detected from RCP to ICP. No temporomandibular joint signs were noted. There was no masticatory muscle tenderness.

● Intraoral

What are your observations from the intraoral views (Figures 9.1 and 9.3)?

Alistair's soft tissues are healthy with the exception of mild marginal gingivitis related to the incisor teeth. His oral hygiene is fair. The dentition appears caries free. 6 e d c 2 1 are present in each quadrant.

Upper and lower incisors are very mildly crowded and in crossbite. The overbite is average to slightly increased and complete. Upper and lower centrelines are displaced. The buccal segment relationship is Class III bilaterally.

What are the possible causes of the reverse overjet?

These are listed in **Table 9.1**.

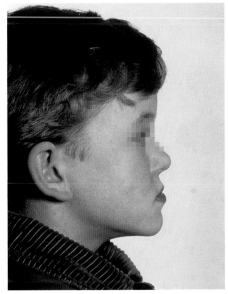

Fig. 9.2 Profile.

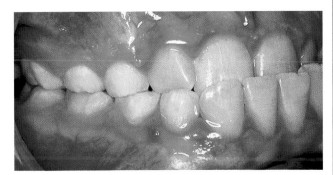

Fig. 9.1 Right buccal occlusion at presentation.

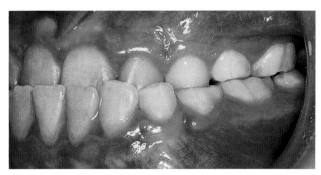

Fig. 9.3 Left buccal occlusion.

Table 9.1 Causes of reverse overjet

Cause	Aetiology
Skeletal	Usually Class III due to any of the following: long mandible, forward placement of glenoid fossa positioning the mandible more anteriorly; short and/or retrognathic maxilla; short anterior cranial base
Anterior mandibular displacement on closure	A premature contact may displace the mandible forward on closure into maximum interdigitation
Retained primary upper incisors	These may deflect the eruption path of their successors palatally into crossbite
Pattern/excessive mandibular growth	Forward pattern of mandibular growth will exacerbate a Class III skeletal pattern. Excessive mandibular growth may be due to excess growth hormone resulting from a pituitary adenoma
Restraint of maxillary growth	Found in repaired cleft lip and palate and attributed to the effect of postsurgical scar tissue

What radiographic investigations would you request and why?

A dental panoramic tomogram would be required to account for all of the remaining permanent teeth.

A lateral cephalometric radiograph is indicated to assess more accurately the magnitude of the Class III skeletal pattern and the incisor angulations, which will facilitate treatment planning. It will also form a baseline from which treatment progress/growth changes can be evaluated by comparison with future cephalometric films.

The panoramic radiograph showed all permanent teeth to be developing.

What is your interpretation of the following cephalometric findings?

SNA = 80°; SNB = 82°; $\underline{1}$ to maxillary plane = 106°; $\overline{1}$ to mandibular plane = 97°; maxillary mandibular planes angle = 25°; Facial % = 53%.

The skeletal pattern is Class III (SNA − SNB = ANB = −2°) due to mild maxillary retrognathism and mandibular prognathism. The upper incisor angulation is within the normal range but slightly retroclined relative to the mean (109°). Taking account of MMPA, $\overline{1}$ angulation should be 120° − 25° = 95°, but is 2° proclined at 97°. The MMPA and facial proportions are slightly reduced from average values but are within the normal range.

Diagnosis
What is your orthodontic diagnosis?

Alistair has a Class III malocclusion on a Class III skeletal pattern with slightly reduced facial proportions. There is an anterior mandibular displacement on closure on $\underline{1|1}$. Upper and lower arches exhibit mild incisor crowding; the upper incisors are in crossbite. The buccal segment relationship is Class III bilaterally.

What is the IOTN DHC score (see p. 183)?

4c due to > 2 mm mandibular displacement between the RCP and ICP.

What dental health reasons are there for orthodontic treatment?

Mandibular displacement on closure may increase the likelihood of temporomandibular joint dysfunction in susceptible individuals. In addition, displacing occlusal contacts may lead to lower incisor mobility and contribute to gingival recession.

What factors would you assess in orthodontic treatment planning?

These are given in **Table 9.2**.

Treatment
What orthodontic treatment would you undertake and why?

In view of the already apparent Class III skeletal pattern, the ability of the patient to just achieve an edge-to-edge incisor relationship, the inherent tendency for downward and forward mandibular growth and the family history, a sensible option would be to accept the malocclusion for the present and reassess in the light of further mandibular growth. Alistair has not yet entered the pubertal growth spurt, which is likely to exacerbate the Class III malocclusion and chin prominence as mandibular growth proceeds. On average, mandibular growth continues until 19 years in boys, but it may progress for longer.

Table 9.2 Factors to assess in treatment planning

Factor	
Degree of anteroposterior and vertical skeletal discrepancy	Most important factor Reflected directly in facial and dental appearance; patient's perception of these will influence complexity of treatment undertaken
Potential direction and extent of future facial growth	Assess relevant family history, age and gender of the patient and vertical facial proportions Reverse overjet is likely to worsen with a forward growth rotation and horizontal pattern of mandibular growth, usually observed when the anterior face height is reduced or average. The converse is likely where there is an increased vertical face height
Incisor inclinations	If dentoalveolar compensation is already marked, further orthodontic compensation is unlikely to be stable or to produce an aesthetic result
Amount of overbite	The deeper the overbite, the better the likelihood of stable correction of the reverse overjet
Ability to achieve edge-to-edge incisor contact	If this is not possible, correction of the incisor relationship by simple means is unlikely
Degree of upper and lower arch crowding	Delay upper arch extractions until the reverse overjet is corrected as this may provide space for relief of mild/moderate crowding If extractions are undertaken in the upper arch only, the reverse overjet may worsen by the upper labial segment moving palatally If mid upper arch extractions are necessary, extraction of $\overline{4|4}$ is usually advisable to allow correction of the incisor relationship

Key point

● Class III malocclusion in the mixed dentition is likely to worsen with mandibular growth, especially in boys.

As the parents are keen for treatment if possible, to try to reduce any further teasing at school, another option to consider would be growth modification by functional appliance therapy (Fränkel III; **Fig. 9.4**) to correct the incisor relationship because:

The skeletal pattern is mildly Class III.

There is an anterior mandibular displacement on closure, i.e. Alistair can achieve edge-to-edge incisor contact.

The MMPA is slightly reduced.

The upper incisors are not proclined.

The lower incisors are very mildly proclined.

The overbite is average to slightly increased.

It is essential, however, that Alistair and his parents are aware of the need for prolonged retention during continuing growth and of the need for reassessment in the light of ensuing growth. This form of treatment should only be undertaken by a specialist and only when Alistair's oral hygiene has improved.

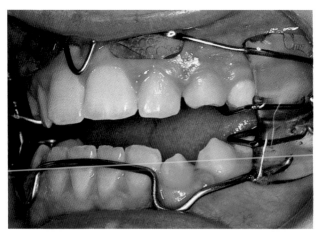

Fig. 9.4 Fränkel III appliance.

How would you take a wax registration for this appliance?

The mandible is rotated downward and backward until the incisors are brought to an end-to-end relationship or better, with the bite open about 2 mm. Alistair can be instructed to place the tip of the tongue at the back of the hard palate and to maintain it there while closing slowly into a horseshoe of softened wax placed over the upper teeth until the desired position is reached. This wax registration should then be chilled in cold water and its accuracy rechecked in the mouth before forwarding to the laboratory with impressions of the dental arches to allow appliance construction.

How much should Alistair wear this appliance?

He should build up wear over the first week so that it is worn for at least 14 hours out of 24. Encouragement should be given to increasing wear to full-time with the exception of mealtimes and for sports, although this may prove difficult for some children. As its name implies, the Function Regulator was designed with the intention of altering function of the circumoral and masticatory musculature. For this reason, the patient should be instructed to 'exercise' these muscles, by gently opening and closing into the appliance. A time sheet should be given to Alistair to allow him to record the number of hours wear per day. This should be inspected at each visit and used to encourage progress.

What effects will this appliance have?

The response is a downward and backward rotation of the mandible accompanied by an increase in facial height. There is no direct restraining force on the mandible and overall attempts to modify growth in Class III cases have proved disappointing. The lower incisors are uprighted and the upper incisors may be proclined slightly. The upper molars should erupt more than the lowers.

> ### Key point
>
> Attempts to 'modify' growth in Class III malocclusion:
> - Tend to be disappointing.
> - Are mostly limited to dentoalveolar changes.

What other treatment options are there?

An alternative approach to try to modify growth where mandibular excess exists is by chin cup therapy. This requires specialist management. The line of force application should be oriented below the condyle to produce downward and backward rotation of the chin. As a result, lower anterior facial height is increased but chin prominence is reduced simultaneously. In essence, the appliance works in exactly the same way as functional appliances for mandibular prognathism. As a significant amount of force from the chin cup is transferred to the base of the lower alveolar process, the lower incisors are also uprighted.

If the patient is not keen to try growth modification or the parents express concern about the need for prolonged retention of the corrected incisor relationship, the malocclusion should be accepted for the present. Arrangements should be made to review occlusal development and to monitor facial growth. In Alistair's case it would be wise to review his occlusion in 18 months (at age 10 years) to check particularly on the position of the unerupted permanent maxillary canines and to measure the reverse overjet.

Once the permanent dentition is established, provided the reverse overjet has not worsened markedly and the chin prominence has not increased greatly, consideration could be given to removal of $\overline{4|4}$ only, in conjunction with upper and lower fixed appliance therapy to correct the incisor relationship. If the upper arch is crowded, $5|5$ may be removed also, but it is wise to delay the decision regarding the need for any upper arch extractions until the reverse overjet has been corrected. It is important to assess the pattern of mandibular growth from an updated cephalometric radiograph prior to this treatment approach, and if there is any concern about it, treatment should be delayed until growth is almost complete.

If the reverse overjet increases considerably with further growth, a combined orthodontic and surgical approach may be required for correction, depending on the patient's concerns. This treatment would not be undertaken until mandibular growth is complete in the late teens.

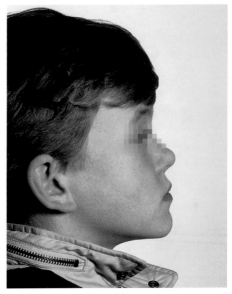

Fig. 9.5 Post-treatment. (a) Profile.

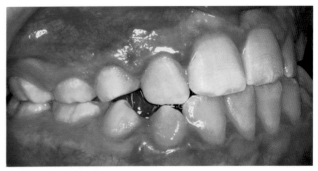

Fig. 9.5 (b) Occlusion.

Prognosis

What factors will influence stability of the corrected incisor relationship?

The amount of overbite is important in the short term but the pattern of facial growth, in particular the magnitude and direction of mandibular growth, will influence longer-term stability.

The profile and occlusion following crossbite correction are shown in **Figure 9.5**.

Recommended reading

Battagel JM 1993 The aetiological factors in Class III malocclusion. Eur J Orthod 15:347–370.

Miethke R-R, Lindenau S, Dietrich K 2003 The effect of Fränkel's function regulator type III on the apical base. Eur J Orthod 25:311–318.

Ülgen M, Firatli A 1994 The effects of the Fränkel's function regulator on the Class III malocclusion. Am J Orthod Dentofacial Orthop 105:561–567.

For revision see Mind Map 9, page 155

10

Increased overbite

Summary

Harry, aged ten and a half, presents with crowded upper teeth and a deep traumatic overbite (**Fig. 10.1**). What has caused these problems and how may they be treated?

History

● Complaint

Harry does not like the appearance of his upper teeth and has recently complained about the gum behind his upper front teeth being sore. His mother is keen for treatment.

● History of complaint

His primary teeth were mildly irregular. His permanent upper front teeth erupted in a 'crooked' position and have not changed since.

● Medical history

Harry is fit and well.

● Dental history

Harry is a regular attender at his general dental practitioner and has not required any dental treatment so far.

● Family history

Harry's father has the same arrangement of the upper anterior teeth as his son. He had four teeth removed and treatment with fixed appliances as a teenager. However, the treatment result relapsed and the upper front teeth

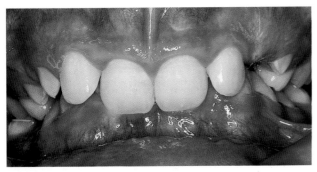

Fig. 10.1 Anterior occlusion at presentation.

have largely returned to their original position. His mother is keen that this does not happen to her son.

Examination

● Extraoral

Harry's profile view is shown in **Figure 10.2.** *What do you notice about the anteroposterior skeletal pattern and the lips?*

Harry has a Class II skeletal pattern with slightly reduced FMPA.

The lips are competent.

● Intraoral

The appearance of the mouth is shown in **Figures 10.1** *and* **10.3.** *What do you see?*

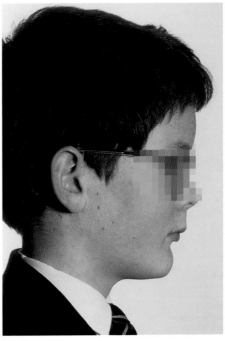

Fig. 10.2 Profile at presentation.

Soft tissues appear healthy apart from mild marginal gingivitis related to the upper incisors.

The oral hygiene is fair with no visible carious lesions.

There are no restorations visible.

Harry is in the mixed dentition with the following teeth visible: $\frac{6\,e\,4\,3\,2\,1\ \ 1\,2\,4\,e\,6}{6\,e\,4\,3\ \ 3\,4\,5\,6}$ ($\overline{2\,1|1\,2}$ are erupted but covered by the upper incisors).

Mild upper labial segment crowding.

Class II division 2 malocclusion with deep complete overbite.

Buccal segment relationships are a half-unit Class II bilaterally.

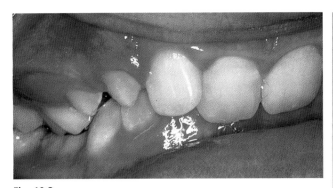

Fig. 10.3 a

Fig. 10.3 b

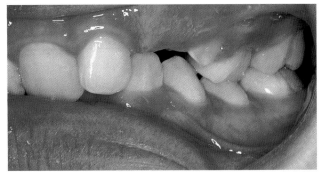

Fig. 10.3 (a) Right buccal occlusion. (b) Left buccal occlusion.

Table 10.1 Causes of increased and traumatic overbite in Class II division 2 malocclusion

Cause	Aetiology
Skeletal: anteroposterior and vertical	A Class II skeletal pattern in combination with a reduced lower facial height
Growth pattern	An anterior mandibular growth rotation tends to increase overbite
Soft tissues	Effects are via the skeletal pattern—reduced lower facial height leads to a high lower lip line that will retrocline the upper incisors, leading to overbite increase A hyperactive high lower lip in association with a reduced lower facial height leads to bimaxillary retroclination
Dental factors	Absence of a well-defined cingulum stop on the upper incisors leads to continued eruption of the lower incisors, increasing overbite

What are the possible causes of the traumatic overbite?

In a Class II division 2 malocclusion several factors contribute to an increased overbite. These are listed in **Table 10.1**.

What further investigations would you undertake?

1. *Assessment of the extent of soft tissue trauma palatal to the upper incisors and labial to the lower incisors from the increased overbite.*

Periodontal pocket depth should be probed in these areas and gingival recession should be noted. Incisor mobility should also be assessed.

Although there was evidence of tooth impingement on the gingivae palatal to $\underline{1|1}$ and labial to $\overline{1|}$, periodontal probing depths did not exceed 2 mm and there was no incisor mobility.

2. *Assessment of the amount of upper and lower arch crowding.* Space to relieve mild/moderate lower arch crowding and level an increased curve of Spee may be obtained by some proclination of the lower labial segment and by a small amount of intercanine width expansion, which appear to be stable in this malocclusion. Therefore, in Class II division 2 malocclusion, lower arch extractions should generally only be undertaken if crowding is severe. In this case, lower arch extractions should be considered with great reservation as this will

allow the lower labial segment to drop lingually and aggravate an already traumatic overbite. There was 2 mm of lower labial segment crowding and space analysis indicated sufficient space for the canines and premolars (21 mm present in each quadrant; 21 mm is required, on average, to accommodate $\overline{3}, \overline{4}, \overline{5}$).

Key point

In Class II division 2 malocclusion:
- Beware of lower arch extractions only, as a deep overbite may become traumatic.
- Some proclination of $\overline{2\,1|\,1\,2}$ and mild lower intercanine expansion are often possible and stable.

3. *Radiographic investigations.* The following views are required:
   (a) Dental panoramic tomogram, to account for the presence/absence, position, form of all unerupted teeth. This showed:
   Normal alveolar bone height.
   Normal developing dentition with a full complement of teeth. No tooth appeared to be in an ectopic position or to be of abnormal size or shape.
   (b) A lateral cephalometric radiograph to assess the anteroposterior and vertical skeletal

relationships and the inclination of the incisor teeth to their underlying dental bases.

What is your interpretation of the following cephalometric findings (see p. 185)?

SNA = 81°; SNB = 74°; ANB = 7°; MMPA = 22°; 1 to maxillary plane = 99°; 1̄ to mandibular plane = 88°; interincisal angle = 162°; Facial % = 51%.

This indicates SNA is average; SNB is reduced; ANB is reduced, indicating a Class II skeletal pattern; MMPA is reduced, which in conjunction with the Class II skeletal pattern is contributing to the increased overbite; 1 to maxillary plane is retroclined; 1̄ to mandibular plane is retroclined, and not compensating completely for the reduced MMPA; interincisal angle is increased; Facial % is reduced.

What is your diagnosis?

Class II division 2 malocclusion in the late mixed dentition on a Class II skeletal base with reduced FMPA and lower facial height. Mild marginal gingivitis related to the upper incisors. Traumatic overbite onto gingivae palatal to 1|1 and labial of 1̄|̄ . Mild upper and lower arch crowding. Buccal segment relationship half-unit Class II bilaterally.

What is the IOTN DHC grade (see p. 183)?

4f due to the traumatic overbite.

Treatment
What are your aims of treatment?

Aims of treatment are to:
Relieve upper arch crowding.
Reduce the overbite.
Correct the incisor relationship to Class I.
Correct the molar relationship to Class I.
Retain the corrected occlusion.

How do you propose to achieve these aims?

As Harry is growing and has Class II and deep bite skeletal problems, growth modification by a functional appliance would be the treatment of choice. A preliminary phase of upper removable appliance therapy will be required to align 1|1 by proclination and to expand the upper arch slightly, allowing the mandible to be postured forward with the arch widths coordinated for the construction bite for the functional appliance. Following that treatment phase, final detailing of the occlusion with fixed appliances is likely to be required prior to proceeding to retention.

Describe the design of appliances you would use

The upper removable appliance to procline 1|1 would have the following components:

Z springs to 1|1 (0.5 mm stainless steel wire).
Midline expansion screw.
Adams clasps 64|6 (0.7 mm stainless steel wire). 4| is insufficiently erupted at present to clasp.
Full palatal acrylic coverage with flat anterior biteplane, initially to half the height of 1|1. A measurement of the overjet plus 3 mm should be forwarded to the laboratory at the time of appliance construction to ensure adequate posterior extension of the biteplane.

As treatment progresses, addition of cold-wire acrylic to the flat anterior biteplane can be made at the chairside, until sufficient overbite reduction has been achieved. The upper incisor teeth should be overproclined slightly to allow for some retroclination under the influence of the functional appliance.

The patient should be instructed to turn the midline expansion screw one quarter turn per week. Arch coordination should be monitored at each recall by getting the patient to posture the mandible foward until the molars are in a Class I relationship and checking to ensure that the buccal segment teeth are not in crossbite. As the upper arch in Class II Division 2 malocclusion is usually square-shaped and the lower arch is 'u'-shaped, only a small amount of upper arch expansion is usually required to achieve coordination of the arch widths with the mandible postured forward.

An activator–bionator type functional appliance is particularly useful in this type of patient. A Herbst appliance is usually not recommended as it tends to depress upper molars and inhibit correction of the deep bite problem. For this case, the construction bite for the activator appliance should be taken with the mandible postured forward edge-to-edge with the incisors apart 3–4 mm and the centrelines correct. If the centrelines had been discrepant by several millimetres initially, the bite should not compensate for this.

The design of a medium opening activator to be used here would be as follows:
Adams clasps and occlusal rests to 6|6 (0.8 mm stainless steel wire).
Labial bow 3| to |3 (0.8 mm stainless steel wire); palatal bow 2| to |2 (0.8 mm stainless steel wire).
Acrylic palatal baseplate, deep acrylic capping of the lower incisors and canines with acrylic struts joining the upper to the lower part of the appliance. The acrylic should be heat-cured.

An alternative to using an upper removable appliance to procline the upper incisors, followed by an activator type appliance, is to use a modified Twin-Block appliance to achieve the desired tooth movements. The design of this appliance incorporates Z springs to procline 1|1, and has no labial bow.

What are the goals of the functional appliance treatment?

To correct the skeletal Class II problem by differential growth of the jaws, in particular addressing the mandibular retrusion.

To increase the lower face height and to correct the deep bite by preventing incisor eruption, controlling eruption of the upper posterior teeth while allowing eruption of the lower posterior teeth. This differential control of incisor/molar eruption aims to rotate the occlusal plane in a manner that allows Class II correction.

Key point

Class II division 2 malocclusion in the mixed dentition may be amenable to functional appliance correction, taking advantage of facial growth to aid overbite reduction.

Why may a later phase of fixed appliance therapy be required?

Rotational correction, especially of 2|2, and detailing of the buccal segment occlusion require the use of fixed appliance therapy.

What aspects of the corrected occlusion are prone to relapse? How may you try to prevent/minimize relapse?

Rotations of 2|2—pericision (severing of the free gingival fibres) should be undertaken a few months prior to fixed appliance removal as it reduces relapse tendency. A bonded retainer, however, will be required to maintain upper labial segment alignment long term.

Overbite—the tendency for anterior mandibular growth rotation to continue into late teens and beyond will encourage overbite increase. To combat this, a flat anterior biteplane should be incorporated on an upper Hawley retainer (designed to fit around the upper bonded retainer) to be worn at night until growth has reduced to adult levels.

Key point

The corrected aspects of Class II division 2 malocclusion most prone to relapse are:
● Rotational correction of 2|2
● Overbite reduction.

The facial profile and the occlusion after functional appliance followed by fixed appliance therapy are shown in **Figure 10.4**.

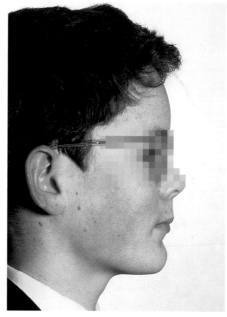

Fig. 10.4 a

Fig. 10.4 b

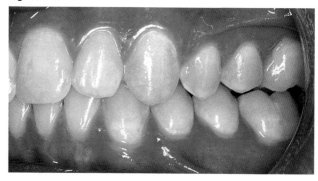

Fig. 10.4 c

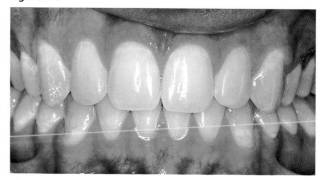

Fig. 10.4 Post-treatment. (a) Profile. (b,c) Occlusion.

Recommended reading

Dyer FM, McKeown HF, Sandler PJ 2001 The modified twin block appliance in the treatment of Class II division 2 malocclusions. J Orthod 28:271–280.

Kim T-W, Little RM 1999 Postretention assessment of deep overbite correction in Class II division 2 malocclusion. Angle Orthod 69:175–186.

Lapatki BS, Mager AS, Schute-Moenting, Jones IE 2002 The importance of the level of the lip line and resting lip pressure in Class II division 2 malocclusion. J Dent Res 81:323–328.

Selwyn-Barnett BJ 1996 Class II division 2 malocclusion: a method of planning and treatment. Br J Orthod 23:29–36.

For revision see Mind Map 10, page 156

Anterior open bite

Summary

Gerald is 11. He presents with no contact of his incisor teeth (**Fig. 11.1**). Identify the cause(s) and discuss the treatment options.

History
● Complaint

Gerald complains that his front teeth do not meet. This embarrasses him when eating as he cannot bite into food. His parents are also concerned by this and by lisping during speech, which they attribute to the position of his front teeth. They are anxious for treatment.

● History of complaint

Gerald's parents report that his primary incisors did not meet either, but the space between the upper and lower permanent incisors appears to have increased in the past year. His lisp has also become more noticeable. He has no history of thumb or digit sucking.

● Medical history

Gerald is fit and well.

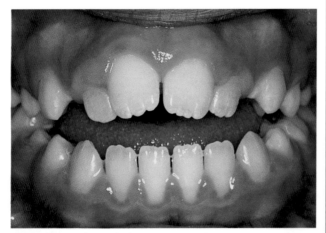

Fig. 11.1 Anterior occlusion at presentation.

● Dental history

Gerald is a regular attender at his general dental practitioner and has cooperated well with previous dental treatment.

Examination
● Extraoral
Gerald's facial profile is shown in **Figure 11.2.** *What do you notice?*

Gerald has a mild Class II skeletal pattern with increased FMPA and increased lower anterior facial height. The lips are competent.

There was no facial asymmetry. Mouth opening was within normal dimensions and there was no temporomandibular joint tenderness or crepitus. No masticatory muscle tenderness was noted.

What other features should you assess? Explain why

1. *The swallowing pattern.* Where there is a space between the upper and lower anterior teeth, swallowing is likely to be achieved by forward positioning of the tongue between the anterior teeth to achieve an oral seal. This is particularly so where the vertical facial proportions are increased as the likelihood of lip incompetence is greater. Although such behaviour of the tongue is in most cases adaptive, in rare instances an endogenous (primary) tongue thrust exists. It has been suggested that this is associated with lisping and some proclination of the upper and lower incisors. Any attempt in these cases to close the open bite is

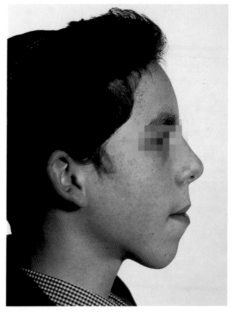

Fig. 11.2 Profile.

doomed to fail as the tongue will return the incisors to their original positions.

2. *Speech.* By asking Gerald to count from 60 to 70 aloud or to say 'Mississippi', the degree of sibilance (lisping) can be detected. The tongue position during speech should also be observed.

Gerald had a tongue to lower lip swallowing pattern and the lisp was deemed to be mild.

What occlusal anomalies are associated with speech problems? Are the latter likely to resolve if any underlying malocclusion is treated?

Although speech problems are associated with incisor spacing, Class II division 1 malocclusion, Class III malocclusion and anterior open bite, they do not occur in all individuals with these occlusal anomalies. Furthermore, correction of these problems is no guarantee that the associated speech problem will resolve satisfactorily. Where sigmatism is judged to be marked, referral to a speech therapist would be prudent, although treatment may do little to mitigate the defect.

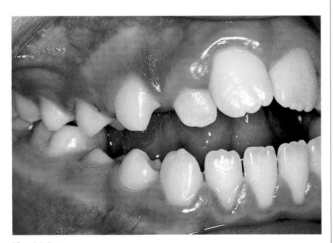

Fig. 11.3 a

Fig. 11.3 b

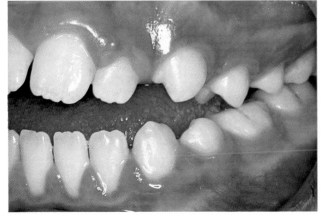

Fig. 11.3 (a) Right buccal occlusion. (b) Left buccal occlusion.

● **Intraoral**
What other features do you see (Figs 11.1 and 11.3)?

Mild marginal gingivitis related especially to the incisors and $4|$.

The dentition is caries free.

Mild spacing of the upper and lower labial segments; mesiolabial rotations of $1|1$.

Class I incisor relationship.

Anterior open bite (measured clinically = 5 mm from the mesio-incisal aspects of $\left|\frac{1}{1}\right.$).

Class III molar relationship bilaterally.

What are the possible causes of an anterior open bite?

These are given in **Table 11.1**.

Table 11.1 Causes of anterior open bite

Cause	Aetiology
Skeletal	Increase in lower anterior facial height such that the compensatory ability of the incisors to erupt into contact is exceeded. This may be worsened by a downward and backward pattern of facial growth
Soft tissues	Rarely endogenous tongue thrust
Habits	Persistent digit-sucking habit, which often leads to an asymmetric anterior open bite
Localized failure of alveolar development	Occurs in cleft lip and palate, although in other cases there may be no known cause

Key point

● A persistent digit-sucking habit often produces an asymmetric anterior open bite.

What are the effects of a persistent digit-sucking habit on the occlusion other than creating an anterior open bite?

It may retrocline the lower incisors, procline the upper incisors, increase the overjet and create a unilateral buccal segment crossbite with associated mandibular displacement (see Chapter 12).

Investigations
What special investigations would you require? Explain why.

A *dental panoramic tomogram* is required to indicate what other teeth have yet to erupt and to check their developmental position and size.

A lateral cephalometric radiograph is required to assess more fully the extent of the anteroposterior and vertical skeletal discrepancies as well as the relationship of the incisors to the underlying dental bases.

The dental panoramic tomogram showed:
Normal alveolar base height.
A normal dentition. The developmental age matches Gerald's chronological age.
Third molars are present.
The cephalometric analysis revealed:

SNA = 82°; SNB = 76°; ANB = 6°; MMPA = 34°; $\underline{1}$ to maxillary plane = 111°; $\overline{1}$ to mandibular plane = 86°; interincisal angle = 126°; Facial % = 60%.

What is your interpretation of these findings?

SNA and SNB are within the normal range for Caucasians; the skeletal pattern is mildly Class II; $\underline{1}$ to maxillary plane is within the normal range; $\overline{1}$ to mandibular plane is compensatory for the MMPA; interincisal angle is reduced but within the normal range; facial proportion is increased.

Diagnosis
What is your diagnosis?

Class I malocclusion on a mild Class II skeletal base with increased FMPA. Marginal gingivitis related to the incisors and $\underline{4|}$. Mild mesolabial rotations of $\underline{1|1}$ with spacing of the upper and lower labial segments. Anterior open bite. Buccal segment relationship Class III bilaterally.

What is the IOTN DHC grade (see p. 183)?

4e due to the anterior open bite.

Treatment
What treatment would you consider?

As the anterior open bite is not due to digit sucking treatment is likely to be complex. Gerald has anteroposterior and vertical skeletal problems, the latter being more marked, with a downward and backward pattern of facial growth that has produced the anterior open bite. An *attempt*, therefore, to achieve incisor contact may be by growth modification aiming for effective control of maxillary vertical skeletal and dental growth.

This would require specialist care. A functional appliance with posterior bite blocks, e.g. a Twin-Block appliance, would be optimal. As the incisor relationship is Class I and the molar relationships are Class III, no forward posturing of the mandible for the registration bite is advisable. The bite, however, must be opened beyond the normal resting vertical dimension so that molar eruption is prevented. As the appliance holds the mandible in this position, a vertical intrusive force is

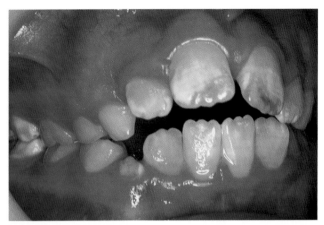

Fig. 11.4 a

Fig. 11.4 b

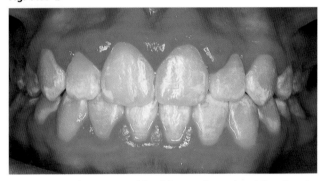

Fig. 11.4 Another case with: (a) anterior open bite due to thumb sucking; (b) following cessation of the habit and fixed appliance therapy.

exerted on the posterior teeth mediated by the stretch of the muscles and other soft tissues. Gerald should be instructed to wear the appliance full-time including for meals. The anterior teeth are allowed to erupt while eruption of the posterior teeth is inhibited, thereby reducing the anterior open bite. This is supplemented by a tendency for mandibular growth to be projected anteriorly while vertical control of maxillary skeletal and dental growth is effected. In this case, high-pull headgear should not be added to the appliance. As the molar relationships are Class III, any molar distal movement is

> ### Key point
>
> ● Unless anterior open bite is due to a habit, treatment is complex.

not indicated.

If the anterior open bite had been due to thumb sucking, what treatment would you recommend?

Gentle persuasion to discontinue the habit is usually best (**Fig. 11.4**). If unsuccessful, consideration could be given to provision of a habit-breaker such as an upper the habit ceases, the anterior open bite will usually reduce spontaneously, although this is likely to take several years.

What is the likely prognosis of treatment?

As the anterior open bite is quite marked and the vertical skeletal pattern is moderately increased, the prognosis is guarded. The parents and child should be made aware of this before treatment commences. Provided there is excellent cooperation with appliance wear and vertical facial growth is favourable, functional appliance treatment has a reasonable chance of success at this stage. However, a second phase of treatment with fixed appliances is likely to be required to detail the occlusion. As these appliances do not control eruption so favourably, posterior bite blocks or similar components will be required during that phase of treatment as well, to maintain the correction achieved in the earlier phase. Thereafter, bite blocks will also need to be incorporated in any retainer. Long-term retention will be required to avert the possible unfavourable effects of subsequent vertical facial growth.

The lisp may improve with closure of the anterior open bite, but Gerald and his parents should not have elevated expectations regarding this.

Are there any other treatment options?

If Gerald does not cooperate with functional appliance wear, treatment for the anterior open bite may be considered by a specific type of fixed appliance mechanics (Kim mechanics), most likely in conjunction with the removal of second or third molars. This approach to appliance treatment requires specialist training. The objective is to correct the cant of individual occlusal planes, uprighting the teeth in relation to the bisecting occlusal plane. Impressive and stable correction of marked anterior open bite, in adolescents and adults, has been reported using this technique. Should the anterior open bite worsen considerably, a combined orthodontic surgical approach may be sought when growth is complete.

Key point

Management options for anterior open bite may be:
- Accept.
- Habit breaker.
- Growth modification.
- Orthodontic camouflage.
- Surgery.

Recommended reading

Johnson NCL, Sandy JR 1999 Tooth position and speech—is there a relationship? Angle Orthod 69:306–310.

Kim YH 1987 Anterior openbite and its treatment by means of multiloop edgewise archwire. Angle Orthod 57; 290–321.

Lopez-Gavito G, Wallen TR, Little RM, Joondeph DR 1985 Anterior open bite malocclusion: a longitudinal 10-year post-retention evaluation of orthodontically treated patients. Am J Orthod 87:175–186.

Mizrahi E 1978 A review of anterior open bite. Br J Orthod 5:21–27.

For revision see Mind Map 11, page 157

Summary

Kirsten is 7. She presents with a crossbite of the right buccal segments (**Fig. 12.1**). What will be your assessment and management options for this problem?

History

● Complaint

Kirsten's mother is concerned about the way her daughter's teeth bite together. She has noticed that Kirsten's jaw moves to one side as she closes her mouth. This makes her face appear crooked, a further cause of anxiety for her mother.

● History of complaint

Kirsten used to suck her thumb until 5 months ago when $\overline{1|1}$ started to erupt. Her mother has become more aware of her daughter's 'deviated bite' in the past year and wondered if the thumb-sucking habit could have contributed to the problem.

● Medical history

Kirsten is fit and well.

● Family history

There is no family history of facial asymmetry.

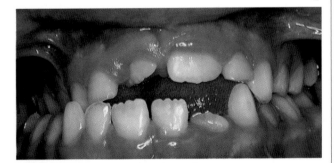

Fig. 12.1 Anterior occlusion at presentation.

Examination

● Extraoral

Kirsten has a mild Class III skeletal pattern with slightly increased FMPA; the chin point is displaced slightly to the right. The lips are incompetent but habitually held together. There is a tongue to lower lip swallowing pattern. There is no masticatory muscle tenderness, temporomandibular joint tenderness or crepitus, and mouth opening is not restricted.

What other feature would you check for, bearing in mind the history? Explain why

It would be important to detect if there is a mandibular displacement on closure as this would indicate that the facial asymmetry is apparent rather than a true skeletal asymmetry. For the former, orthodontic correction of an associated crossbite should be straightforward but for the latter further investigations would be required to determine if the asymmetry is progressive and more complex treatment would be required to address the facial and occlusal problems.

Early correction of a crossbite with a mandibular displacement is indicated to allow the occlusion to develop in an undisplaced position. It is likely also to reduce the possibility of development of temporomandibular joint dysfunction syndrome, which may occur in susceptible individuals where this occlusal discrepancy exists.

An anterolateral mandibular displacement on closure was detected on $\frac{c|}{c|}$ with an associated 3 mm shift between retruded contact position (RCP) and intercuspal position (ICP).

Key point

Early correction of a posterior crossbite with associated mandibular displacement is advisable.

● Intraoral
What features are evident on the intraoral views (Figs 12.1 and 12.2)?

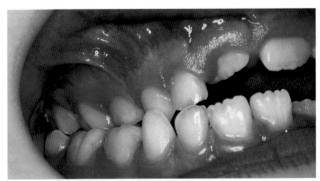

Fig. 12.2 a

Fig. 12.2 b

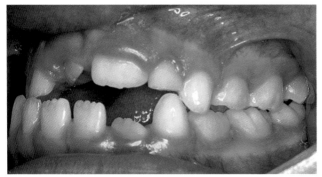

Fig. 12.2 (a) Right buccal occlusion. (b) Left buccal occlusion.

Mild marginal gingival erythema related to the erupting permanent incisors but otherwise the soft tissues appear healthy.

Spacing of the upper and lower incisors with distopalatal rotation of 1| .

Class III incisor relationship.

Lower centreline shift to the right.

Anterior open bite.

Half-unit Class II right molar relationship with buccal crossbite of the right buccal segments (note palatal inclination of the teeth).

Class III left molar relationship.

How would you assess the centrelines?

The upper and lower centrelines should be coincident with each other and with the midline of the face. Both of these aspects should be assessed, the latter by first looking at the patient anteriorly and then down on the face from above. With study models alone, it is not possible to determine the relation of the incisor midlines to the facial midline.

In this case, the lower centreline is displaced to the right by half the width of a lower incisor.

Box 12.1 Causes of a lower midline shift

- Unbalanced loss of c, d and possibly e; the age at extraction, the degree of crowding and the tooth extracted (the more anterior, the greater the effect) influence the extent of centreline shift.
- Unilateral retained primary incisor, canine or molar
- Hypodontia of an incisor or premolar
- Supplemental incisor or premolar
- Lateral mandibular displacement on closure producing unilateral buccal segment crossbite (often secondary to digit- or thumb-sucking habit)
- Early unilateral condylar fracture leading to deficient growth on the affected side
- Hemifacial microsomia
- Hemimandibular hypertrophy (known formally as condylar hyperplasia). Cause is entirely unknown. Most likely in females between the ages of 15 and 20 but may occur in either sex as late as the early thirties

What are the possible causes of a lower centreline shift?

These are listed in **Box 12.1**. In this case, it is due to the lateral mandibular displacement on closure.

What factors may be implicated in the aetiology of the crossbite?

These are summarized in **Table 12.1**.

Table 12.1 Causes of buccal segment crossbite

Cause	Aetiology
Skeletal	Mismatch in the widths of the dental arches and/or an anteroposterior skeletal discrepancy—buccal and anterior crossbites are most commonly found in Class III cases. Rarely, mandibular growth restriction following condylar trauma or condylar hyperplasia may be implicated, both producing asymmetry
Soft tissues/habit	With a digit-sucking habit, the tongue position is lowered with the teeth apart, and cheek contraction is unopposed during sucking, narrowing the upper arch slightly.

What is the most likely cause of the posterior crossbite in this case?

The thumb-sucking habit.

Key point

A digit-sucking habit may lead to posterior crossbite with associated mandibular displacement.

Investigation
What special investigations would you undertake and why?

A dental panoramic tomogram (**Fig. 12.3a**) is required to survey the developing dentition for any abnormalities of tooth number, size and position.

Impressions of the dental arches and a wax registration in maximum intercuspation should be taken to allow study models to be made. These will allow a thorough occlusal assessment to be performed and will act as a baseline record of the occlusion.

What does the dental panoramic tomogram show?

Normal alveolar bone height.

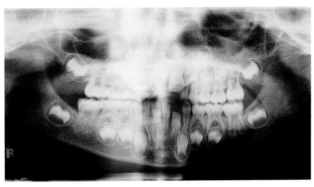

Fig. 12.3 a

Fig. 12.3 b

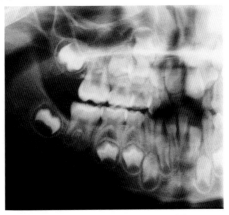

Fig. 12.3 (a) Dental panoramic tomogram. (b) Repeat of right half dental panoramic tomogram.

All permanent teeth developing apart from third molars.

No apparent caries or other pathology.

What is the most likely reason for the blurred image of the right half of the dental panoramic tomogram?

Movement of the patient during image capture, most probably due to swallowing, is the likely cause.

Why was a right half, rather than a full, dental panoramic tomogram retaken? (Fig. 12.3b)?

In line with current radiology guidelines, the radiation dosage to the patient should be as low as reasonably achievable for the diagnostic purposes required. Retaking the right-half image only satisfies diagnostic needs here.

Diagnosis
What is your diagnosis?

Class III malocclusion on a Class III skeletal base with slightly increased FMPA. Mild marginal gingivitis related to the erupting incisors. Spacing of the upper and lower incisors with $\underline{1|}$ distopalatally rotated. Anterior open bite; lower centreline shift to the right. Buccal segment relationship half-unit Class II on the right and Class III on the left. Buccal crossbite of the right buccal segments with associated mandibular displacement on closure.

What is the IOTN DHC grade?

4c due to mandibular displacement > 2 mm between the RCP and the ICP.

Treatment
What treatment plan would you propose?

Oral hygiene instruction to improve gingival health.
Correction of the right buccal segment and anterior crossbites.
Regular review of the developing occlusion.

How may the crossbites be corrected? Describe the design of any appliance you would use

Possible approaches to treatment are as follows:

1. As the digit-sucking habit has been abandoned and the mandibular displacement arises from premature contact on $\frac{c|}{c|}$, judicious grinding of their cusp tips may remove the occlusal interference and correct the buccal segment crossbite. A systematic review on management of posterior crossbites concluded that removal of premature displacing contacts on primary teeth prevents perpetuation of the posterior crossbite into the permanent dentition. The permanent incisors are erupted insufficiently, at present, to consider their proclination and which means will be best.

2. As the upper buccal segment teeth are not tilted buccally, upper arch expansion by a midline screw in an upper removable appliance may be considered. The appliance may be clasped on $\underline{6\,d|d\,6}$. Buccal capping will facilitate tooth movement by disengaging the posterior occlusion. Kirsten should be encouraged to turn the screw one quarter turn twice weekly (0.25 mm of activation with each turn) until the crossbite is corrected. A small amount of overexpansion is advisable as some relapse is to be expected. Then the capping should be reduced to half its height at one visit and removed completely at the following visit to allow the buccal segment teeth to erupt into occlusion. The appliance should then be worn for 3 months full-time followed by 3 months at night only as a retainer.

3. Alternatively, upper arch expansion may be undertaken using a quadhelix. This consists of bands cemented to the first permanent molars with soldered arms, in this case, extending forward to the palatal aspects of $\underline{c}$'s. Alternatively, a preformed quadhelix may be employed that fits

into sheaths soldered to molar bands, allowing easy removal for adjustment. Activation is usually 1 cm on each side in the molar region and about 1.5 cm in total in the anterior region. To facilitate crossbite correction, it may be necessary to disengage the buccal occlusion by placing glass ionomer cement on the occlusal surfaces of the molars. Once the crossbite has been corrected, the quadhelix should be rendered passive prior to cementation for 3–6 months as a retainer. Research has shown that the expansion achieved by an upper removable or a quadhelix appliance is similar but the latter is more cost-effective.

The final occlusion following crossbite correction by an upper removable appliance is shown in **Figure 12.4**.

Correction of the incisor relationship and improvement in $\underline{1|}$ alignment occurred spontaneously.

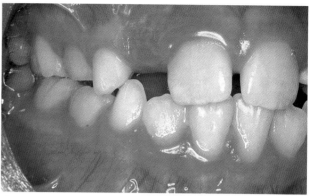
Fig. 12.4 a

Fig. 12.4 b

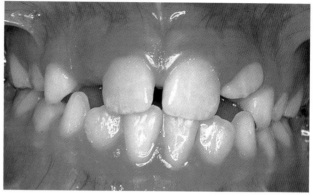
Fig. 12.4 (a,b) Post-treatment.

Key point

Management options for a unilateral posterior crossbite with associated mandibular displacement in the mixed dentition:
- Grind c's.
- URA with midline screw.
- Quadhelix.

What will determine if the corrected buccal segment crossbite is likely to be stable?

Good buccal segment interdigitation and absence of any displacing occlusal contacts are required.

Recommended reading

Harrison J, Ashby D 2004 Orthodontic treatment for posterior crossbites. Cochrane Review. The Cochrane Library, Issue 24. John Wiley, Chichester.

Hermanson H, Kurol J, Ronnerman A 1985 Treatment of unilateral posterior crossbites with quadhelix and removable plates. A retrospective study. Eur J Orthod 7:97–102.

For revision see Mind Map 12, page 158

13

Late lower incisor crowding

Summary

Graham is almost 20 years old. He presents with crowding of his lower incisors (**Fig. 13.1**). What is the cause and how would you treat it?

History

● Complaint

Graham is concerned about the crowding of his lower front teeth and wonders if it will get worse.

● History of complaint

His lower front teeth were straight until 18 months ago when he noticed crowding developing. He now finds it more difficult to keep his lower front teeth clean. Calculus build-up also seems to occur more easily on the inside of the lower teeth, which he finds annoying. He is also aware of two wisdom teeth erupting at the back of his lower jaw for the past 18 months. These do not cause him any problems but he wonders if they are making his lower front teeth crooked.

● Medical history

Graham is fit and well.

● Dental history

Two years ago previously, he had a course of fixed appliance therapy, to close a large space between $1|1$ followed by composite build-up of $2|2$.

Examination

● Extraoral examination

Graham has a Class I skeletal pattern with average FMPA and no facial asymmetry. Lips are competent. There are no signs or symptoms associated with the temporomandibular joints.

● Intraoral examination

The appearance of the teeth on presentation is shown in **Figures 13.1 and 13.2**.

What do you notice?

Lower labial segment crowding with $\overline{8|8}$ erupting.
Class I incisor relationship, although it appears to be tending towards Class III.
Right buccal segment relationship Class III.

Is lower incisor crowding common at this age?

In the late teens, it is very common in modern populations for crowding to develop of the mandibular incisor teeth. This strong tendency occurs even if the teeth were well aligned or spaced initially, leading usually to mild crowding, whereas initial mild crowding tends to become worse. Lower labial segment crowding also occurs where extractions for relief of crowding and fixed appliance therapy have been undertaken (unless a bonded lingual retainer has been placed).

What are the possible causes of late lower incisor crowding?

The aetiology is multifactorial and the major theories proposed are as follows:

1. *Late mandibular growth.* Forward mandibular growth, especially if a growth rotation is also present, and where maxillary growth has stopped, aided by lip pressure, tends to reposition the lower

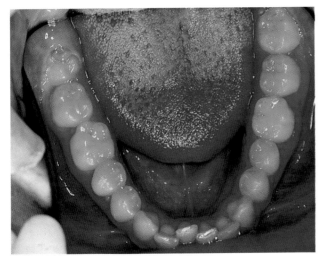

Fig. 13.1 Lower occlusal view at presentation.

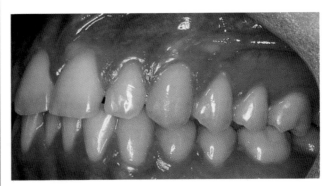

Fig. 13.2 Right buccal occlusion.

incisors lingually, reducing arch length and causing anterior crowding. Currently it is thought that as the lower incisors and maybe the whole lower dentition move posteriorly relative to the mandibular body late in mandibular growth, lower incisor crowding almost always develops. The greater the magnitude of late mandibular growth when other growth has essentially stopped, the greater the likelihood of developing late lower incisor crowding. On average, in a male patient, as is the case here, mandibular growth is complete by 19 years but it may continue for longer.

2. *Gingival and/or occlusal forces.* Pressure from the transseptal fibres and/or the anteriorly directed component of occlusal forces lead to mesial migration of the dentition.

3. *Lack of approximal attrition in modern diet.* This was thought to explain absence of lower labial segment crowding in Australian Aborigines but has not been borne out by research findings.

4. *Reduction in intercanine width.* After age 9, the mandibular intercanine width reduces gradually during teenage years, and this progresses at a reduced rate into adult life. The result is an increase in lower labial segment crowding, most marked during late teens.

5. *The presence of third molars.* Their role is controversial. Two theories abound:
   (a) They may exert mesial pressure on the lower dentition during eruption, tending to produce lower labial segment crowding.
   (b) They may prevent the lower teeth from moving distally in response to forces generated by mandibular growth or soft tissues.

However, late lower incisor crowding develops even when third molars are absent so their presence is not the critical factor in the aetiology of the problem. The amount of late mandibular growth is paramount.

Key point

Possible factors in the aetiology of late lower incisor crowding include:
- Late mandibular growth.
- Gingival and/or occlusal forces.
- Reduction in intercanine width.
- Third molars?

Investigations
What investigations would you undertake? Explain why

1. *Radiographic.* A dental panoramic tomogram would be useful to assess the position and inclination of the partially erupted lower third molars. As a radiograph was taken prior to commencing orthodontic treatment, this should be consulted first and the need for a further radiograph should be assessed based on the clinical assessment and the radiographic findings.

2. *Study models.* Upper and lower impressions and a wax registration in centric occlusion should be taken for study models to record accurately the current malocclusion and to allow further treatment planning.

What do you notice on the dental panoramic tomogram taken pre-orthodontic treatment (Fig. 13.3)?

Normal alveolar bone height.
All teeth present and of good quality.
$\overline{8|}$ slightly mesioangularly impacted.
$\overline{8|}$ upright (bone overlies the distal half of the crown of both lower third molars).

Diagnosis
What is your diagnosis?

Class I malocclusion with late lower incisor crowding on a Class I skeletal pattern with average FMPA; right buccal segment relationship Class III; impacted lower third molars.

What are the management options for late lower incisor crowding?

1. *Accept and monitor.* As this is a normal maturational change in the lower arch, it would be sensible in a late teenager, and where the crowding is mild, to keep it under observation. Where more marked crowding is present, intervention can be considered.

2. *Interproximal stripping.* This is only acceptable in an adult with mild lower incisor crowding. By removing 0.25 mm at most from the mesial and

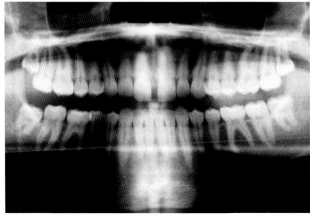

Fig. 13.3 Dental panoramic tomogram.

distal aspects of each incisor, up to 2 mm of space can be obtained for relief of crowding. Incisor alignment may then be achieved by a localized fixed appliance. A removable appliance, with an acrylated labial bow or Invisalign® (a clear polyester-based appliance) made to fit a duplicate study model with the incisors aligned with their mesial and distal surfaces reduced, are alternative approaches. With Invisalign®, however, several appliances may be required to achieve incremental change until the final alignment has been realized. A bonded retainer will be required to maintain the result long term.

3. *Extraction of a lower incisor.* Where the lower labial crowding is marked, removal of a lower incisor may be indicated to give sufficient space for alignment of the remaining units. It is advisable to carry out a diagnostic wax-up on a duplicate set of study models to ascertain what the final result is likely to be and to ensure the patient is happy with this before proceeding with the extraction. The patient should be warned of the possibility of the upper labial segment moving palatally, with resultant misalignment, in response to the lower labial segment being aligned slightly lingually. Unless the incisor to be extracted is completely excluded from the arch and the remaining incisors are well aligned, fixed appliance therapy is inevitably indicated to detail the position of the remaining labial segment teeth. Bonded lingual retention will then be required.

4. *Extraction of lower premolars.* Where the buccal segment occlusion is well interdigitated and crowding is confined to the lower labial segment, it is preferable to avoid lower mid-arch extractions because these will disrupt the buccal occlusion. Instead removal of a lower incisor will expedite lower labial segment alignment while preserving the integrity of the buccal segments.

Would you advise removal of the lower third molars?

Lower third molars should not be removed in an attempt to prevent further increase in lower labial segment crowding, as their relation to this aspect of malocclusion is unproven.

Current guidelines advise removal of lower third molars only if they are associated with recurrent episodes of pericoronitis or other pathology. In this case, as neither of these apply at present, the lower third molars should be retained and their position reviewed if symptoms develop.

Key point

Management options for late lower incisor crowding:
- Accept and monitor.
- Interproximal stripping with appliance therapy.
- Lower incisor extraction with appliance therapy.

How would you manage the lower incisor crowding?

Monitor the eruption of the lower third molars.

As the lower labial segment crowding is mild to moderate, advise Graham to accept it for the present. It should be kept under review and if the crowding increases, then consideration could be given to treatment.

Recommended reading

Dacre JT 1985 The long-term effects of one lower incisor extraction. Eur J Orthod 7:136–144.

Harradine NWT, Pearson MH, Toth B 1998 The effect of extraction of third molars on late lower incisor crowding: a randomized controlled trial. Br J Orthod 25:117–122.

Little RM, Reidel RA, Årtun J 1988 An evaluation of changes in mandibular anterior alignment from 10 to 20 years post retention. Am J Orthod Dentofacial Orthop 93:423–428.

NHS Centre for Reviews and Dissemination, York 1999 Prophylactic removal of impacted third molars: is it justified? Br J Orthod 26:149–151.

Richardson ME 2002 Late lower arch crowding: the aetiology reviewed Dent Update 19:234–238.

For revision see Mind Map 13, page 159

14

Prominent chin and TMJDS

Summary

Jocelyn, aged 23, is referred by her general dental practitioner regarding her prominent chin and pain in her left TMJ (**Fig. 14.1**). What are the causes and how would you manage these problems?

History

● Complaint

Jocelyn's main concern is that she does not like the prominent appearance of her chin and her upper teeth biting inside her lower teeth. She has pain in her left jaw joint and has some difficulty chewing. She is also aware that she has a lisp, which she dislikes.

● History of complaint

Jocelyn has been aware of her prominent chin and her bite for the past 5 years. After consultation with an orthodontist at age 12, she had upper first premolars removed to provide space for the upper eye teeth. (The

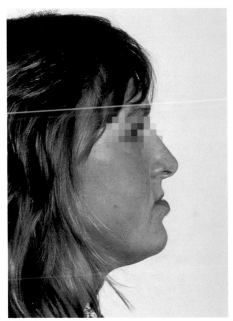

Fig. 14.1 Profile at presentation.

lower permanent molars had been extracted at age 8 because of decay.) She did not wear any braces on her teeth. She was advised to wait until she was in her late teens to have the bite of her front teeth reassessed. In the past 6 months she has become quite self-conscious about her facial appearance, although she feels that her chin does not appear to have become more prominent in the past 4 years.

What questions would you ask about the temporomandibular joint pain?

When it started; how it started; type of pain; duration.
Frequency.
Is it localized? Site of radiation.
Associated symptoms, e.g. muscle pain, click, jaw locking, trismus.
Aggravating factors, e.g. stress.
Any habits, e.g. nail biting, bruxism, pen chewing.
Relieving factors, e.g. heat, analgesics (type and amount).

The pain started suddenly when Jocelyn was preparing for examinations in her first year at university. She has had intermittent discomfort in her left jaw joint for the past 6 years but it has been of a mild nature. The discomfort is an ache that is principally in the left jaw joint area but radiates to the jaw muscles on that side. It does not keep her awake at night but she feels it is worse in the morning. Typically it lasts for a few hours and then disappears. It tends to return when Jocelyn is stressed by work. She is aware of grinding her teeth when stressed. She does not engage in chewing pencils or pens or nail biting. She feels that in the past year the pain has recurred more frequently and has become worse. Chewing hard food or opening her mouth too wide makes the pain worse; one or two paracetamol tablets usually relieves the ache. Jocelyn is also aware that she has a jaw click.

● Medical history

The patient is fit and well.

● Dental history

Jocelyn is a regular attender at her general dental practitioner and brushes twice daily.

● Family history

Jocelyn's sister also has a prominent chin, but not as marked as hers, and her sister's bite was corrected with fixed braces.

Examination

● Extraoral examination

What do you observe from Jocelyn's profile view (Fig. 14.1)?

Class III skeletal pattern with average FMPA.
Competent lips.

Based on the history, what other aspects would you assess extraorally?

The temporomandibular joints. Opening and lateral mandibular movements should be assessed by first observing the patient from in front and second by palpation of the condylar heads while listening for the presence of crepitus or a joint click. As symptoms are present, the masticatory muscles should also be palpated. A left TMJ click and left masseteric tenderness were detected.

The mandibular path of closure. The path of closure from rest position to maximum interdigitation should be assessed, noting any anterior or lateral mandibular displacement produced by a premature contact.

In this case, there is an anterior mandibular displacement on closure on contact of $\frac{7|}{8|}$ (centric relation to centric occlusion shift ~3 mm).

● **Intraoral examination**

The intraoral views are shown in **Figure 14.2**.

What do you see?

Gingival tissues appear healthy; gingival recession related to $\dfrac{6\ 3\ |\ 3\ 5\ 6}{7\ |}$.

Oral hygiene appears good.

$\dfrac{7\ 6\ 5\ 3\ 2\ 1\ |\ 1\ 2\ 3\ 5\ 6}{8\ 7\ 5\ 4\ 3\ 2\ 1\ |\ 1\ 2\ 3\ 4\ 5\ 7}$ are visible

No obvious caries.

Mild lower incisor crowding with spacing between the $\overline{4}$'s and $\overline{5}$'s.

Mild upper arch crowding with slight mesiolabial rotations of $2|2$.

Class III incisor relationship with reverse overjet (measured 4 mm clinically), reduced overbite and coincident dental centrelines.

Class I canine relationship bilaterally.

Buccal crossbite affecting $\frac{7|}{8|}$.

What is the most likely cause of the considerable spacing in the lower premolar areas with $\overline{5}$'s drifted into contact with $\overline{7}$'s?

Early removal of $\overline{6\ e\ |\ e\ 6}$ in an uncrowded arch is the most likely explanation for the spacing. An uncrowded lower arch is common in Class III malocclusion.

What occlusal features may predispose to temporomandibular joint dysfunction syndrome?

Crossbites, Class III malocclusion and anterior open bite have a statistically significant association with temporomandibular joint dysfunction syndrome (TMJDS) in some

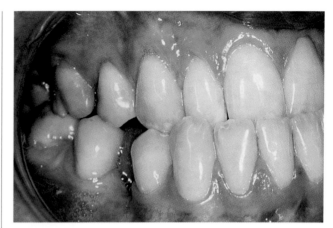

Fig. 14.2 a

Fig. 14.2 b

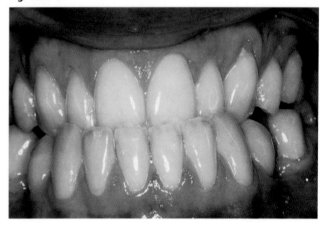

Fig. 14.2 c

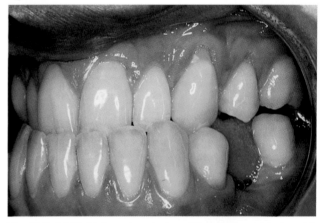

Fig. 14.2 (a) Right buccal occlusion. (b) Anterior occlusion. (c) Left buccal occlusion.

studies while others have found no link between signs and symptoms of TMJDS and mandibular displacements. The aetiology of TMJDS is multifactorial with the implicated involvement of psychological, traumatic and occlusal elements. The most salient factor is probably stress, which may transmit its effect by a parafunctional habit, stemming perhaps from a displacing occlusal contact in susceptible individuals. In this case, a displacement existed on $\frac{7|}{8|}$ on closure. There are also anterior and posterior crossbites present.

Why was Jocelyn advised to wait until her late teens for reassessment?

In a Class III malocclusion, the amount of reverse overjet tends to increase with forward mandibular growth during teenage years. Waiting until mandibular growth is essentially completed, which is generally about 17 years in girls and 19 years in boys, has three advantages. First, it allows treatment planning to be undertaken with reasonably stable facial and occlusal characteristics. Second, if treatment is undertaken, it safeguards against relapse due to further growth. Third, the magnitude of occlusal change due to mandibular growth influences whether treatment can be undertaken by orthodontic means alone or whether a combined surgical–orthodontic approach is necessary. Orthodontic treatment involves inducing dentoalveolar compensation for the underlying skeletal pattern, but if unsuccessful due to continued adverse mandibular growth the compensation would need to be undone as part of presurgical orthodontics. This may involve opening up lower premolar extraction spaces. Hence the decision to treat a Class III malocclusion in early teenage years by orthodontic camouflage that includes lower arch extractions must be made with great caution.

In this case the severity of the anteroposterior skeletal pattern, the likely pattern of mandibular growth, the amount of dentoalveolar compensation, the amount of overbite and the relative absence of crowding would all have been considerations in delaying any orthodontic intervention. Whether the patient could achieve an edge-to-edge incisor relationship would also need to have been assessed.

Key point

Waiting until at least late teens before considering an orthodontic/orthognathic approach is desirable as:
- Facial and occlusal characteristics stabilize.
- It safeguards against relapse due to further growth.
- Camouflage or surgery is determined by the extent of mandibular growth.

Investigations
What investigations are required and why?

The patient's primary concern is about her facial appearance and she has a malocclusion, which is likely to be untreatable by orthodontic means alone. A combined orthodontic–surgical approach is required. The investigations required, in such cases, together with reasons for their selection, are listed in **Table 14.1**. The TMJ assessment has already been undertaken for Jocelyn (p. 59).

The dental panoramic tomogram showed no condylar pathology.

The cephalometric values are as follows:

SNA = 79°; SNB = 85°; ANB = –6°; $\underline{1}$ to maxillary plane = 113°; $\overline{1}$ to mandibular plane = 82°; interincisal angle = 139°; MMPA = 26.5°; SN to maxillary plane = 11°; Facial % = 56%.

What is your interpretation of these findings (see p. 185)?

Moderately severe Class III skeletal pattern due to a combination of maxillary retrognathia and mandibular prognathism. As SNA is 2° less than the mean of 81°, application of the Eastman correction adds 1° to the ANB to give a revised ANB value of –5°.

Slightly proclined upper incisors (although inclination is within the normal range) and markedly retroclined lower incisors indicating dentoalveolar compensation for the Class III skeletal pattern. The lower incisor angulation must be considered with the MMPA—this has been explained on page 31.

Interincisal angle is within the normal range for Caucasians.

MMPA, SN to maxillary plane and Facial % are within the normal range for Caucasians.

Diagnosis
What is your diagnosis?

Class III malocclusion on a Class III skeletal base with average FMPA. TMJDS with left TMJ click. Previous loss of $\overline{6}$'s and $\underline{4}$'s. Very mild lower labial segment crowding. Uncrowded upper arch. All of the upper arch in crossbite with the exception of $\underline{6\ 5\,|\,5\ 6}$. Buccal crossbilte on $\dfrac{7}{8}$ with associate mandibular displacement.

What is the IOTN DHC score?

5m due to reverse overjet greater than 3.5 mm with reported masticatory and speech difficulties.

Treatment
What are the aims of treatment?

Relief of the TMJDS.

Correction of the underlying skeletal Class III problem.

To establish Class I incisor and molar relationships.

To correct the buccal segment crossbites.

To restore the lower buccal segment spaces.

Table 14.1 Investigations required in combined surgical – orthodontic planning

Investigation required	Reason
Thorough clinical assessment of facial form in full face and profile	To locate any cranial, maxillary, nasal, mandibular or chin deformities
	To assess the height and width proportions of the face, interalar distances, nasolabial angle, upper incisor exposure, relation of upper dental midline to other facial midlines, the form and tone of the soft tissues
Assessment of TMJ	To record signs and/or symptoms of TMJ dysfunction. Treat these conservatively if possible prior to treatment; if marked occlusal problems contributing to dysfunction, aim to correct these with treatment
Dental panoramic tomogram (DPT)	To assess the general dental status and prognosis of the dentition as well as the position of unerupted third molars (bitewing or periapical radiographs may be required depending on clinical and/or DPT findings)
Lateral cephalometric radiograph	To ascertain the aetiology of the malocclusion and to facilitate surgical planning
Facial and dental photographs	To record the facial and dental characteristics of the malocclusion
	To allow surgical planning either by enlargement of a negative of the patient's profile to fit 1 : 1 with the lateral cephalometric film or by video-imaging systems
Study models and duplicates mounted on an articulator	To allow thorough orthodontic/occlusal assessment and model surgery

What treatment is required? Explain why

A combined orthodontic–surgical approach is needed due to:

- The patient's concern relating to facial and dental appearance.
- The severity of the underlying Class III skeletal pattern.
- Despite the degree of dentoalveolar compensation, a reverse overjet of 4 mm exists.
- An ANB angle of greater than −4° and lower incisor angulation to the mandibular plane of less than 83° have been found indicative of an orthodontic–surgical approach.

How will this case be managed?

● Short term

A hard full coverage upper acrylic splint should be made and Jocelyn should be instructed to wear this full-time until the TMJ symptoms subside. She should also be advised to take a soft diet and to avoid straining her jaw joints by, e.g. wide yawns. Mild analgesics should also be taken as required.

● Longer term

A combined orthodontic–surgical approach is required to correct the facial and occlusal problems. The TMJDS symptoms may ease with orthodontic treatment. This is due to tooth movement rendering the teeth tender on biting, so parafunctional activity stops because tooth clenching/grinding does not produce the same sub-conscious pleasure as previously. The improvement in symptoms may be transient, even if displacing occlusal contacts (present here on $\frac{7}{8}|$) are eliminated.

The patient should be warned about the unpredictable impact of orthognathic surgery on TMJDS to avoid unreasonable expectations of treatment.

Key point

- Orthodontic treatment and/or orthognathic surgery cannot be guaranteed to eliminate TMJDS.

Explain how you would proceed with surgical planning for this case

1. A team approach is required involving the orthodontist and the oral and maxillofacial surgeon. The input of a restorative specialist is also required in relation to management of the lower premolar spacing. Jocelyn must understand that to obtain the best facial and occlusal result possible, fixed appliance therapy is essential to the overall plan.
2. Surgical planning may be undertaken by various means. After tracing or digitizing the patient's cephalometric film, a 'standard' skull template (e.g. Bolton standard representing the norm) may be superimposed on it to indicate sites of discrepancy. These templates, however, are composites of males and females. Alternatively,

enlargement of a negative of the patient's profile photographic view to fit 1 : 1 with the lateral cephalometric film, followed by a process of 'cutting and pasting' to simulate the desired surgical changes, may be undertaken. Both of these methods are tedious and a simpler more efficient means is via a computer program that allows movements to be planned and displayed visually on a screen before printing.

3. Video-imaging techniques also allow superimposition of the patient's profile on the cephalometric tracing. The video image is adjusted in line with changes in the tracing, allowing the patient to visualize the anticipated surgical outcome. Using reference lines to measure distances, planned surgical movements should then be transferred to a duplicate set of study models, mounted on a semiadjustable articulator in this case as maxillary surgery is planned.

4. The final plan should be explained to Jocelyn, ensuring that she is aware that her profile will be worsened by presurgical orthodontics and that she realizes what her final facial appearance is likely to be. If she wishes, arrangements should be made for her to meet and discuss the process with another patient for whom a successful outcome was achieved.

Key point

Planning surgical–orthodontic treatment:
- Requires a team approach.
- May be assisted by:
  matching facial photographs and radiographs
  computer programs
  video-imaging.

Describe the phase of presurgical orthodontics

This phase of fixed appliance treatment aims to allow the jaws to be moved to their desired location without interference from tooth positions. The upper and lower arches are aligned and coordinated as well as establishing the vertical and anteroposterior position of the incisors. This involves decompensating for any existing dentoalveolar compensation. In this case this will involve primarily labial movement of the lower incisors, which will eliminate the mild crowding and slight uprighting of the upper incisors. The full extent of the skeletal discrepancy is thus revealed, maximizing the extent of possible surgical correction. Class II intermaxillary traction may be required to aid decompensation. No extractions are indicated in this case to achieve the desired tooth movements. The gingival status labial to the

lower incisors should be monitored during decompensation to ensure that gingival recession does not ensue.

When the requisite tooth movements have been achieved, rigid rectangular stainless steel archwires should be used to passively stabilize tooth position. Final presurgical records—study models, photographs and a cephalometric film—will then be taken to assess the changes that have occurred and to decide if the original surgical plan will be followed or require some amendment. Hooks should be attached to the archwires just prior to surgery. These facilitate intermaxillary fixation and/or elastic traction postoperatively.

Key point

Presurgical orthodontics:
- May involve extractions.
- Usually decompensate for any dentoalveolar compensation.
- Align and coordinate arches or arch segments.
- Establish the vertical and anteroposterior position of the incisors.
- Place rigid rectangular archwires with ball-hooks immediately presurgically.

What surgical procedures are likely to be required?

- Le Fort I advancement.
- Mandibular setback.

What form of splint and fixation is likely to be required?

An interocclusal acrylic wafer, fabricated to fit articulator mounted casts positioned to the desired occlusal result, is recommended routinely to ensure accuracy of the postsurgical result. Following Le Fort I advancement and mandibular setback osteotomies, mini-plates and lag screws are likely to be required respectively for fixation. Intermaxillary fixation may also be required. If not and a jaw exercise programme is commenced immediately after surgery, mouth opening will be satisfactory 2–3 weeks later. This will allow the use of light elastic traction to guide jaw function while maintaining the acrylic splint in place to key the occlusion.

Describe the postsurgical orthodontic phase

When a satisfactory range of mandibular movement and stability of the osteotomy sites have been achieved, the acrylic splint should be removed. Light round archwires should be placed immediately to allow occlusal settling, often aided by the use of posterior box elastics with an anterior force vector, which helps maintain the sagittal corrections. When good interdigitation has been achieved, elastic wear should be discontinued. Rarely will this phase of treatment take longer than 6 months to complete. A period of retention is then required, no different to that for other adults. Surgical follow-up should be for a minimum of 2 years.

What factors influence post-surgical stability?

Stability will be influenced by:

Orthodontic and surgical plans being correct, realistic, well-integrated and undertaken competently.

Modest surgical movement—no greater than 6 mm in any direction in the maxilla or 8 mm in the mandible—does not place the soft tissues under tension and the condyles are not distracted at surgery.

Absence of tongue thrust, previous surgical scarring.

Patient compliance with all aspects of treatment, particularly postsurgical wear of elastic traction.

Adequate fixation.

The postsurgical profile and occlusion are shown in **Figure 14.3**.

Key point

● Stability is enhanced when surgical movement is modest and does not induce soft tissue tension.

Recommended reading

Hunt NP, Rudge SJ 1984 Facial profile and orthognathic surgery. Br J Orthod 11:126–136.

Luther F 1998 Orthodontics and the temperomandibular joint: where are we now? Angle Orthod 68:295–318.

Proffitt W, White R, Sarver D 2003 Contemporary treatment of dentofacial deformity. Mosby, St Louis.

For revision see Mind Map 14, page 160

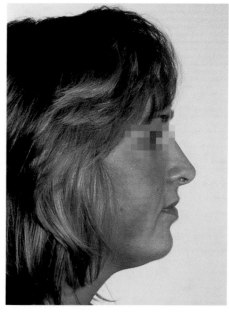

Fig. 14.3 a

Fig. 14.3 b

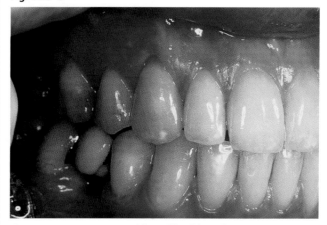

Fig. 14.3 Post-treatment. (a) Profile. (b) Occlusion.

15
Drifting incisors

Summary

Iain, a 51-year-old male, presents with spacing and mobility of his upper incisors (**Fig. 15.1**). What is the cause and what can be done?

History
● Complaint

Iain complains of the spacing of his upper incisors and looseness of these teeth, particularly of $2|$ and $\overline{|2}$. He is self-conscious of the upper anterior spacing and is worried in case the incisors fall out.

● History of complaint

He has noticed increasing mobility of his upper front teeth over the past few months. The spacing between the teeth appeared at the same time and is becoming progressively worse. There is no pain associated with the mobility of the teeth but eating has become uncomfortable. He is also aware of mobility of his lower incisors and of several upper and lower posterior teeth. Recently he has experienced an unpleasant taste in his mouth, which appears to originate from the upper front teeth.

● Dental history

Iain has been a regular attender at another dental practice for many years, before moving to your area. He is

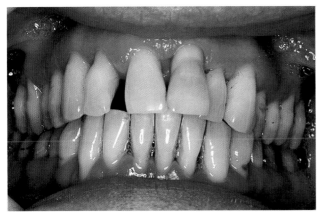

Fig. 15.1 Occlusion at presentation.

highly motivated and does not wish any tooth to be lost. $|1$ was traumatized in his early twenties and has become progressively darker but he is unconcerned by this.

● Medical history

Iain is an insulin-controlled diabetic. He is otherwise fit and well.

● Social history

He smokes 10 cigarettes a day and has done so for 30 years.

Examination
● Extraoral

There are no palpable submandibular or cervical lymph nodes.

● Intraoral
What do you notice in Figure 15.2?

Oral hygiene appears good with generalized interproximal staining. Gingivae related to the lower incisors appear oedematous.
Generalized gingival recession.
Heavily restored dentition with $|1$ discoloured.
Mild lower anterior crowding.
Space between $2\ 1|$ and mild crowding $|1\ 2$.
Class III incisor relationship with minimal overbite and overjet except for $2|1$; upper and lower centrelines are not coincident.

Based on what you know so far, what are the possible factors implicated in respect to mobility and drifting of 21|12 ?

Chronic periodontal disease is a definite possibility when the overall periodontal condition is observed.
Periapical periodontitis is another possibility but this would also tend to lead to extrusion of these teeth, which is not markedly evident.
Root resorption. This would have to be extensive to produce such spacing and mobility.
Root fractures. This is not a possibility in view of the history.
Other pathology such as radicular cyst or bony lesions are rarer possibilities.

What would you check for specifically in relation to the history?

Degree of any tooth mobility.
Presence, extent and location of plaque and/or supra-/sub-gingival calculus deposits.
Presence/site of bleeding on probing.
Presence/site of periodontal purulent exudate.
Presence/site of a sinus and/or associated exudate.
Presence/site of any deep carious lesion.
Occlusal factors that may contribute to tooth

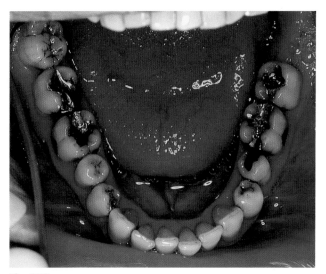

Fig. 15.2 a

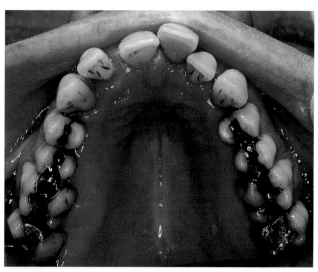

Fig. 15.2 b

Fig. 15.2 c

Fig. 15.2 d

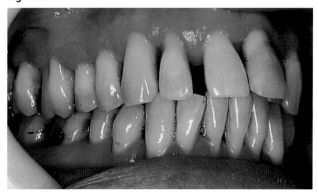

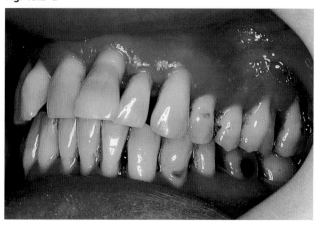

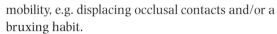

Fig. 15.2 (a) Lower occlusal view. (b) Upper occlusal view. (c) Right buccal occlusion. (d) Left buccal occlusion.

mobility, e.g. displacing occlusal contacts and/or a bruxing habit.

Other habits, e.g. pen chewing, nail biting.

Calculus is present subgingivally on all teeth with generalized 4–6 mm pocketing and delayed bleeding on probing. There is a purulent discharge from the periodontal pocket on the mesial aspect of $2\rfloor$. No sinuses are present. There are no carious teeth.

Upper and lower molars, premolars and canines exhibit Grade I mobility buccolingually but not vertically. Upper and lower incisors have Grade I mobility buccolingually but *not* vertically except for $\overline{2}$ which exhibits Grade II mobility buccolingually and vertically.

Iain has right and left group function in lateral excursions. There are no occlusal interferences in protrusion.

Investigations
What other investigations would you carry out? Why?

Full-mouth periapical radiographs are required to assess accurately the periodontal status, particularly the alveolar bone height as well as the presence of any periapical pathology.

Full-mouth radiographs are shown in Figure 15.3. What do you see?

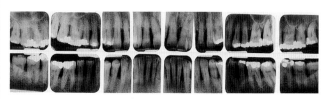

Fig. 15.3 Full-mouth periapical radiographs.

Generalized horizontal bone loss of at least 50% with angular bone defects affecting $\dfrac{2\mid 1}{6\ 3\mid 2\ 6}$.

70–80% alveolar bone loss affecting the lower incisor teeth.

Heavily restored dentition but no caries visible.

Diagnosis
What is your diagnosis?

Chronic moderate periodontitis with localized areas of advanced disease. Class III malocclusion with mild lower incisor crowding and spacing/drifting of the upper incisors.

With loss of periodontal attachment, how may labial drifting of the incisors occur?

Alveolar bone loss compromises the ability of the teeth to deal with soft tissue and occlusal forces, thereby leading to tooth movement.

A traumatic occlusion may result from extrusion as a consequence of periodontal inflammation. Drifting may occur where periodontal support is also reduced.

Labial shift of periodontally involved upper incisors may result also from a displacing occlusal contact on closure producing a forward mandibular slide.

Undue forces may be placed on the incisors, where posterior tooth support is lacking due to tooth loss, and these can lead to upper incisor proclination.

Key point

Migration of periodontally involved incisors may be exacerbated by:
● A forward mandibular displacement on closure.
● Deficient posterior occlusal support.

What is the significance of the medical history and social history to the diagnosis?

Diabetes affects the host response to periodontal pathogens by altering polymorph chemotaxis. Although the diabetes is well controlled in Iain's case, periodontal disease is chronic and generalized due to inadequate oral hygiene measures exacerbated by the host response.

Smoking contributes significantly to periodontal disease through a variety of means. Gingival blood flow is reduced; salivary flow is slowed also, leading to poorer removal of periodontopathic bacteria and encouraging calculus build-up.

Treatment
What treatment would you advise?

Cessation of smoking. The patient should be encouraged to stop smoking to prevent any further insult to his periodontal health imposed by this habit.

Referral for joint periodontal/orthodontic consultation. His condition requires specialist care in view of the advanced nature of the periodontal disease.

What periodontal treatment do you envisage will be required?

Oral hygiene instruction, particularly in the use of interproximal cleaning aids.

Full-mouth scaling and root planing.

Reassessment.

Consider localized surgery to those areas where response to primary phase therapy is inadequate, i.e. bleeding/purulent exudate on probing persists.

How would you describe the prognosis of his dentition?

Prognosis depends on the response to initial therapy and patient factors such as motivation towards maintainence of a very high standard of oral hygiene and cessation of the smoking habit.

Based on the amount of alveolar bone loss, the prognosis of the upper incisors is likely to be better than that of the lower incisors.

What are the treatment options for the upper labial segment spacing?

1. Orthodontic alignment of the upper labial segment teeth with space closure. Six months after completion of periodontal therapy, the periodontist should re-evaluate the periodontal status. Provided it has not deteriorated and Iain is not adverse to the prospect of wearing an orthodontic appliance, orthodontic treatment could be considered.

2. Extraction of $\underline{2|}$ or of $\underline{2\,1|1\,2}$ and replacement on a partial upper denture or adhesive bridgework. Extraction of $\overline{1|1}$ may be required also with similar prosthetic replacement to the extracted upper units.

Iain opted for fixed appliance therapy to align the upper teeth (**Fig. 15.4**).

What special considerations are there with orthodontic treatment in a periodontally compromised dentition?

Bands should be avoided due to the risk of further compromising periodontal support by placement of the band margin subgingivally, creating a nidus for plaque accumulation. Bonded attachments, therefore, should be placed on all teeth including molars.

If several posterior teeth have been lost, anchorage for the tooth movements required may not be sufficient and reinforcement with a bonded transpalatal arch or implant may be necessary.

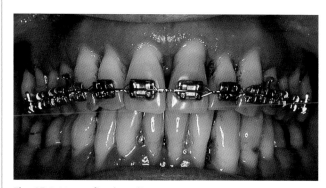

Fig. 15.4 Upper fixed appliance.

With reduced alveolar bone support, light forces should be applied to the teeth.

When gingival recession is evident pretreatment, the patient should be warned as to the possibility of this being aggravated by orthodontic tooth movement.

Regular periodontal recall should be undertaken throughout orthodontic treatment.

Due to loss of periodontal attachment and alveolar bone, permanent bonded retention will be required.

The final occlusion is shown in **Figure 15.5**.

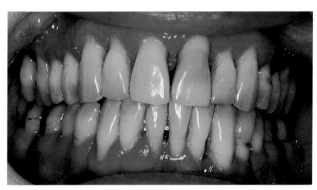

Fig. 15.5 Final occlusion with bonded palatal retainer in place.

Key point

For orthodontic treatment in a periodontally involved dentition:
- Avoid bands.
- Use light forces.
- Ensure regular periodontal recall during treatment.
- Retain permanently.

Recommended readings

Gustke CJ 1999 Treatment of periodontitis in the diabetic patient. A critical review. J Clin Periodontol 26:133–137.

Nattrass C, Sandy JR 1995 Adult orthodontics—a review. Br J Orthod 22:331–337.

For revision see Mind Map 15, page 161

16

Appliance-related problems

Case 1
Summary

Leanne, a 12-year-old girl, presents for a routine check of her upper retainer. You notice a reddened palate (**Fig. 16.1a**). What is your diagnosis and what management would you institute?

History
● Complaint

Leanne's only complaint is that her upper retainer is loose. She is not aware of any problem with her palate.

● History of complaint

Leanne has been wearing the upper removable retainer for the past 10 weeks. 5|5 were absent and she had e|e removed to provide space for relief of upper arch crowding. She was offered upper fixed appliance treatment to produce the best occlusal result but she was not keen for this. Instead, she opted for upper removable appliance therapy. She has worn one previous appliance. The current appliance has been getting progressively looser over the past month.

● Medical history

Leanne is asthmatic and has used a Ventolin inhaler for the past 4 years. Her asthma is well controlled.

Examination
● Extraoral

Leanne has a Class I skeletal pattern with average FMPA and no facial asymmetry. Her lips are competent, with the lower lip just covering the incisal third of the upper anterior teeth. There are no temporomandibular joint signs or symptoms.

● Intraoral

The soft tissues appear normal except for generalized mild marginal gingivitis and the palatal mucosa, which is shown in **Figure 16.1a**. Oral hygiene is fair.

Describe the appearance of the palate

The lesion affecting the palate can be described as follows:

Site—palatal mucosa and attached gingivae.

Size—area affected relates to that covered by the baseplate of the upper removable retainer (**Fig. 16.1b**).

Shape—the posterior limit of the lesion is semilunar and defined, as is the rest of the lesion, by the baseplate outline.

Colour—uniformly reddened appearance of the palate and attached gingiva underlying the baseplate with some petechial areas along the right posterior palatal extension.

Background—mucosa and gingivae not covered by the baseplate appear of normal colour.

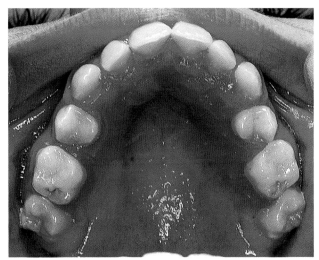

Fig. 16.1 a

Fig. 16.1 b

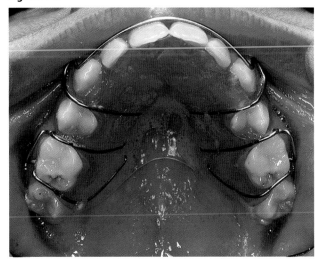

Fig. 16.1 (a) Appearance of the palate at presentation. (b) Upper removable retainer.

What are your observations regarding the retainer?

The appliance is a Hawley retainer with Adams clasps on 6|6 and a labial bow from 3| to |3. The baseplate is made of clear acrylic.

Appliance hygiene does not appear optimal—food debris and plaque deposits are visible, through the baseplate, on the fitting surface of the appliance.

What is the most likely diagnosis based on the information you have so far?

Palatal (denture) stomatitis as it is symptom-free.

What other condition would produce a similar appearance?

Acrylic allergy. This, however, is unlikely as a 'burning' sensation of the mucosa underlying the baseplate would have been reported early after insertion of the first upper removable appliance and there would be erythema of all of the soft tissues adjacent to the acrylic.

What is the aetiology of 'denture' stomatitis?

Candida is the principal cause. Although a normal oral commensal, its proliferation is facilitated by local environmental or systemic factors, thereby allowing it to become pathogenic (**Table 16.1**).

Key point

- Candida is the principal cause of palatal stomatitis related to an upper removable appliance.

What factors in this case may have predisposed to 'denture' stomatitis?

The use of a steroid inhaler, poor appliance hygiene and full-time wear of the appliance are likely to be the main contributory factors. A direct relationship has been shown between the presence of an upper removable appliance, candida and low salivary pH levels. In addition, upper removable appliance therapy has a positive, though transient, influence on the prevalence of candida and density of oral candidal carriage, suggesting that the carrier state may be initiated by the appliance.

Investigations
How would you confirm the diagnosis?

The ideal investigation is a smear from the palatal mucosa underlying the baseplate for microbiological testing.

Saliva sampling for candida counts.

Culturing for accurate identification and sensitivity testing may also be undertaken.

Table 16.1 Causes of denture stomatitis

Factor	Aetiology	
Local	Infection with candida (~90% due to *Candida albicans*) Poor denture/appliance hygiene Night-time wear of denture/appliance Possible trauma Poor salivary clearance of oral commensals High sugar intake providing substrate for candida proliferation	
Systemic	Iron and vitamin deficiencies Steroids Drugs that cause xerostomia Endocrine abnormalities, e.g. diabetes, Antibiotic therapy	predispose to candida infection

What stains identify candida?

Gram stain: candida is strongly Gram positive.

Periodic acid–Schiff (PAS): a magenta stain locates carbohydrate in fungal cell walls.

Treatment
How would you treat this condition?

Leanne should be advised to:

1. Leave the appliance out at night. Timing is fortuitous as she is in the retention phase of treatment, and in 2 weeks time she is due to progress to night-only wear of the retainer. Due to the infection, it would be wise to wear the appliance throughout the day but remove it at night until the palatal mucosa returns to health.
2. Improved appliance hygiene—brush the fitting surface and soak it in a 1% hypochlorite solution.
3. Improve oral hygiene—teeth, gingivae and palatal mucosa should be brushed thoroughly after every meal.
4. Reduce sugar intake—alter diet to a low-carbohydrate consumption.
5. Antifungal agents (nystatin or amphotericin suspension or miconazole oral gel) should be applied to the fitting surface of the appliance four times daily. A 2% chlorhexidine mouthwash may also be beneficial due to its antifungal effect.

As the asthma is well controlled, there is no need to refer Leanne to her general medical practitioner.

Key point

Management of palatal stomatitis:
- Leave appliance out at night.
- Improve appliance hygiene and oral hygiene.
- Reduce carbohydrate consumption.
- Antifungal agents.

What is the prognosis for this condition?

Provided all the above strategies are followed, the condition should resolve completely within a few weeks.

Recommended reading

Arendorf T, Addy M 1985 Candidal carriage and plaque distribution before, during and after removable orthodontic appliance therapy. J Clin Periodont 12:360–368.

Wilson J 1998 The aetiology, diagnosis and management of denture stomatitis. Br Dent J 185:380–384.

Cases 2 and 3
Summary

Two common fixed appliance problems are shown. What is the cause of each and what treatment would you provide?

What problem do you notice in Figure 16.2a?

A bracket has become debonded from $\overline{5|}$.

Why has this occurred?

Bond failure may occur for various reasons (**Table 16.2**).

Treatment
What treatment would you provide? Explain why

The patient should be advised first to contact their orthodontist for repair of the appliance (**Fig. 16.2b, c**).

If this is not possible and the loose bracket is at risk of being swallowed or inhaled, it should be removed. In this case, however, this risk is less likely as the bracket remains attached to a ligature wire and elastometric module.

Should the loose bracket be a source of discomfort to the patient, as a general dental practitioner, you could remove the loose bracket and the loose ligature. The patient should be appointed with their orthodontist at the earliest opportunity.

What problem do you notice in Figure 16.3a?

The cheek mucosa is ulcerated due to trauma from the overextended round archwire.

How has this problem arisen?

The amount of projection of the archwire beyond the molar band may have been overlooked at the time of archwire placement, or the archwire may have moved to its current position following insertion, as the teeth aligned, or due to loss/bond failure of another appliance component.

How would you manage this problem?

As a general dental practitioner, you should, first, advise the patient to contact their orthodontist to deal with this problem. If this is not possible then you should provide emergency care.

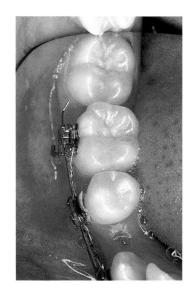

Fig. 16.2 a

Fig. 16.2 b

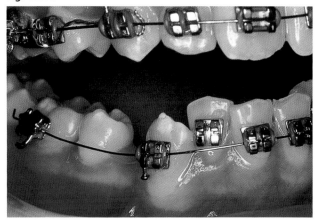

Fig. 16.2 c

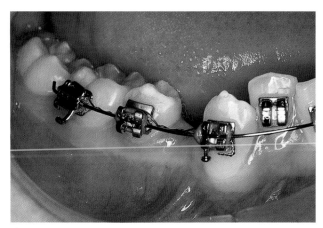

Fig. 16.2 (a) Lower occlusal view. (b) Following removal of ligature wire and $\overline{5|}$ bracket. (c) Following replacement of ligature wire and rebonding of a $\overline{5|}$ bracket.

As a general dental practitioner, what emergency care would you provide?

The distal end of the archwire should be cut flush with the terminal aspect of the molar tube or the archwire end turned underneath the molar tube or angled inward away from the cheek (**Fig. 16.3b**). As a round nickel

Table 16.2 Causes of bracket bond failure

Factor	Aetiology
Operator	Insufficient etch time
	Poor etch pattern[a]
	Poor moisture control during bonding
	Non-adherence to manufacturer's instructions with the bonding adhesive chosen
	Movement of the bracket after initial placement, which interferes with bond formation within the adhesive
	Application of high force to the bracket to accomplish archwire engagement
Patient	Eating hard/sticky foods
	Possibly use of phenolic-containing mouthrinses that soften composite
	Occlusal trauma/bruxing habit
	Pen chewing/nail biting

[a] Etch pattern is poorer on premolars than on canine or incisor teeth. This contributes to the greater bond failure rate on premolars (note failure in Fig. 16.2a is on 5̅|).

titanium wire is in place, with the terminal end heat-treated (note blackened appearance), this is easily cut to the desired length or positioned to avoid cheek trauma.

The patient should be advised to maintain a high standard of oral hygiene and to rinse with lukewarm salty water after meals until the ulceration heals. Provision of a supply of soft wax to apply over the molar tube and the adjusted wire end may also be helpful in the intervening period. The patient should also schedule an appointment in the near future with their orthodontist.

Key point

Emergency treatment for:
- Loose bracket: remove if risk of ingestion/inhalation.
- Overextended archwire: cut wire and/or turn wire end inward away from the cheek.

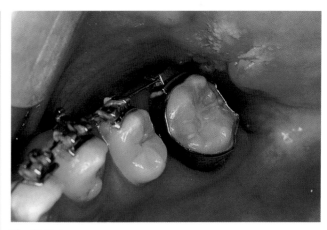

Fig. 16.3 a

Fig. 16.3 b

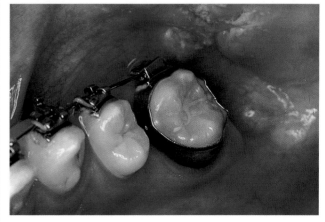

Fig. 16.3 (a) Upper occlusal view. (b) Following shortening and adjustment of upper archwire.

Recommended reading

Hobson RS, Rugg-Gunn AJ, Booth TA 2002 Acid-etch patterns on the buccal surface of human permanent teeth. Arch Oral Biol 47:407–412.

Mandall NA, Millett DT, Mattick CR, Hickman J, Worthington HV, Macfarlane TV 2002 Orthodontic adhesives: a systematic review. J Orthod 29:205–210.

For revision see Mind Map 16, page 162

17

Tooth movement and related problems

Case 1
Summary

Darren, a 13-year-old boy, has been undergoing upper removable appliance therapy to retract and align 3| for 6 months, following extraction of 4| . Tooth movement has been very slow with no movement recorded at the last two visits.

What are the possible reasons for a slow rate of tooth movement?

These can be divided broadly into patient, appliance and operator factors.

● Patient factors

The patient is not complying with appliance wear as instructed.
Incorrect positioning of the spring on appliance insertion or distortion of the spring.
Contact of the tooth with the buccal cortical plate or with a retained root part of 4| .
The occlusion with the opposing arch may prevent tooth movement.

● Appliance factors

Acrylic and/or wire may be interfering with tooth movement.

● Operator factors

Design flaws, underactivation, overactivation or activation of the spring such that 3| is directly buccally into contact with the cortical plate rather than through the cancellous corridor of bone.

What force range is optimal for retraction of 3| by tipping movement?

The optimal force range is 30–50 g or 0.3–0.5 N.

What cellular response is there following activation of the spring to retract 3| by tipping movement?

The consequence of the spring activation is the setting up of pressure and tension zones within the periodontal ligament. Half of the periodontal ligament is stressed with maximum pressure created at the alveolar crest in the direction of movement and at the diagonally opposite apical area (**Fig. 17.1**)

Key point

● Tipping movement, typically, requires forces of 30–50 g or 0.3–0.5 N.

● Pressure zones

The cellular response depends on whether a light or heavy force is applied. With a light sustained force, tooth movement occurs within a few seconds as periodontal ligament fluid is squeezed out and the vascular supply is compressed, setting off a complex biochemical response. Within 2 days, osteoclast invasion occurs and frontal resorption follows.

When a heavy sustained force is applied, the periodontal ligament is compressed to such a degree that the blood supply is cut off completely, producing an area of sterile necrosis (hyalinization). Small areas of hyalinization are inevitable even with light forces, but the area of hyalinization is extended with forces of greater magnitude. Osteoclast differentiation is impossible within the necrotic periodontal ligament space, but after several days osteoclasts appear adjacent to and within the adjacent cancellous spaces. From there they invade the bone adjacent to the hyalinized area and tooth movement eventually occurs by undermining resorption.

● Tension zones

Following initial application of a light force, the blood vessels vasodilate and the periodontal ligament fibres are stretched, while fibroblast and preosteoblast proliferation

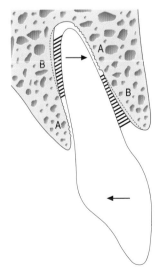

Fig. 17.1 Diagram to illustrate zones of pressure (A) and tension (B) in the periodontal ligament induced by a tipping force.

occurs. The stretched fibres become embedded in osteoid, which later mineralizes. The normal periodontal ligament width is eventually regained by simultaneous collagen fibre remodelling.

With heavy forces, rupture of blood vessels and severing of the periodontal ligament fibres are likely but these are restored with the remodelling processes.

Key point

- Application of a sustained force to a tooth creates areas of pressure and tension within the periodontal ligament, which ultimately lead to bone resorption and deposition respectively.

What is the mechanism for tooth movement?

Although the histological response to an applied orthodontic force has been investigated extensively, the mechanism by which a mechanical stimulus is transferred to a cellular response is complex and is at present unresolved. It is likely that vascular changes in the periodontal ligament in areas of pressure and tension, electrical signals in response to alveolar bone flexing following force application, as well as prostaglandins and cytokine release interact in the process.

How would you manage the problem in this case?

Management is specific to each cause. The action taken may be one or more of the following:

The need for full-time wear of the appliance must be emphasized to the patient/parent. They must be made aware that treatment will be ceased unless full cooperation is forthcoming.

Show the patient how to insert the appliance with the spring positioned correctly and explain the action of the spring. Ensure that the appliance is not being removed by the spring.

Check the activation of the spring and adjust it appropriately.

Remove any acrylic or wire obstruction to tooth movement. This may involve remaking the appliance to an improved design.

Add to a flat anterior biteplane or buccal capping to disengage the occlusion, if this is hampering tooth movement.

Ask the patient and check their case records regarding any noted problem with the extraction of 4|. If indicated, take a periapical radiograph of 4| extraction site to check for a retained root fragment. If this is detected, seek an oral surgical opinion regarding its removal or whether it could be left in situ and its position monitored radiographically.

Check 3| is not ankylosed. This is unlikely in this case as some movement of 3| has occurred since 4| was extracted.

Darren admitted to intermittent wear of the appliance and, in particular, to leaving it out at meals. He was advised accordingly.

Key point

- Full-time wear of an upper removable appliance is required for an optimal rate of tooth movement.

What do you notice on the periapical radiograph of another case (Fig. 17.2)?

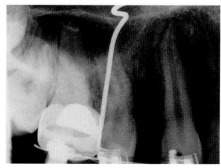

Fig. 17.2 Periapical radiograph

There is a retained small apical root fragment of 4|.

What treatment would you advise?

Complete retraction of 3| is unlikely due to the presence of this root fragment. However, its removal would require a surgical procedure, which would destroy a considerable amount of alveolar bone and may damage the roots of the adjacent teeth. The root fragment may resorb in time and become confluent with the alveolar bone.

In view of the surgical risks, it would be wise to leave the root fragment in situ, monitor its status radiographically and accept the limitation this poses to complete retraction and alignment of 3|.

Recommended reading

Ren Y, Maltha JC, Kuijers-Jagtman AM 2003 Optimum force magnitude for orthodontic tooth movement: a systematic literature review. Angle Orthod 73:86–92.

Roberts-Harry D, Sandy J 2004 Orthodontics. Part II: Orthodontics tooth movement. Br Dent J 196:391–394.

Case 2
Summary

Alan is reviewed 3 months after completion of a 2-year course of upper and lower fixed appliance therapy. He is wearing upper and lower removable retainers full-time.

On removal of the retainers, you detect Grade 2 mobility of the upper incisors and Grade 1 mobility of all other teeth anterior to and including the first permanent molars in both arches. His oral hygiene is good and there is no bleeding on probing. You order a dental panoramic tomogram.

Why is the radiograph ordered?

It will allow a general screen of alveolar bone height and root length of all teeth.

What do you notice on the film (Fig. 17.3a)?

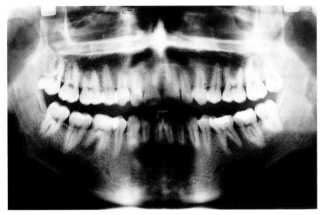

Fig. 17.3 a

Fig. 17.3 b

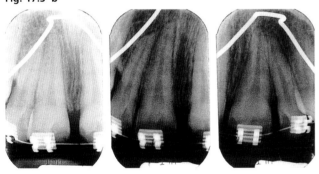

Fig. 17.3 c

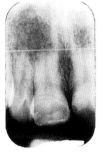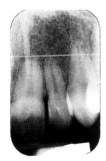

Fig. 17.3 (a) Dental panoramic tomogram. (b) Periapical radiograph of upper incisors taken 6 months into treatment. Note no apical root resorption apparent on |1 2 but slight apical resorption of 2 1| roots. (c) Periapical radiograph indicating marked root resorption of 2 1|1 2 .

Generalized apical blunting (root resorption) of all teeth, anterior to and including the first permanent molars. The upper incisors appear to exhibit most root resorption.

What dental radiographic signs have been shown to predispose to an increased risk of root resorption with orthodontic treatment?

Teeth with pipette-shaped or blunted roots, those which have experienced trauma previously and teeth with short roots and previous root resorption are more susceptible to root resorption with orthodontic forces.

Alan sustained coronal fractures involving enamel and dentin of 1|1 3 months before starting orthodontic treatment.

What other factors have been related to orthodontically induced root resorption?

A strong familial association has been reported.
Patients with chronic asthma, both medicated or non-medicated, have an increased incidence of maxillary molar root resorption.
Invagination and taurodontism have been found to be risk factors.
Extensive apical movement of the roots promotes more marked resorption. No malocclusion, however, is immune to this type of root resorption.

> ### Key point
>
> The risk of orthodontically induced root resorption is increased for teeth with:
> - Pipette-shaped or blunted roots.
> - A history of trauma.
> - Short roots.
> - Previous root resorption.

Could root resorption have been prevented?

Root resorption has a multifactorial aetiology and some amount is regarded as an unavoidable sequela of orthodontic tooth movement. Although, on average 1 mm of root length will typically be lost over a 24-month course of orthodontic treatment, wide individual variation exists. It remains impossible to identify with a degree of certainty an appliance system that will reduce or eliminate apical root resorption.

Aside from evaluating the radiographic and other parameters listed previously, excessive forces and/or too frequent appliance adjustment should be avoided.

Teeth at risk should have a periapical radiograph taken pretreatment and at 6 months into treatment (**Fig. 17.3b**). If apical root resorption is identified then, treatment should be halted for 8–12 weeks with a passive archwire. When severe apical resorption is detected, the treatment goals should be reconsidered with the patient and alternative options explored.

What must the orthodontist ensure before treatment commences?

The risk of apical root resorption as a consequence of orthodontic treatment must be explained to the patient/parents and discussed with them. In addition, an informed consent form signed by patient/parents and the orthodontist must describe, in particular, the risk of apical root resorption. Treatment should not be offered unless the anticipated benefits far outweigh the risk of minor apical resorption seen in most patients.

Appropriate radiographs should be taken including periapical films of teeth at greater risk of apical root resorption, as outlined previously.

Key point

- Root resorption is a common consequence of orthodontic treatment.
- Explain the risk to the patient before treatment starts and obtain consent.
- Monitor radiographically teeth at risk.

What would you do in this case?

Ask the patient if he is aware of marked mobility of any teeth and/or any other symptoms.

Clinically, the mobility of all teeth should be recorded. Alan was aware of upper incisor mobility.

Enquire about bruxism or other habits, such as nail-biting. None were reported.

Sensibility testing of the incisors and canines should be undertaken. All teeth were responsive to sensibility testing and no marked differences in recordings were detected between each tooth and its opposite number in each arch.

What treatment would you provide?

Alan should continue with full-time wear of his retainers for another 3 months and then proceed to night-only wear for at least a further 6 months.

Periapical radiographs should be taken of the upper incisors as these exhibit Grade 2 mobility (**Fig. 17.3c**). Follow-up radiographic examinations and sensibility tests are recommended at 6 months to ascertain if the apical root resorption is progressive. This, however, should be unlikely as 'active' orthodontic treatment has been concluded.

Recommended reading

Al-Qawasmi RA, Hartsfield JK, Everett ET et al 2003 Genetic predisposition to external apical root resorption. Am J Orthod Dentofacial Orthop 123:242–252.

Brezniak N, Wasserstein A 2002 Orthodontically induced inflammatory root resorption. Part I. The basic science aspects; Part II. The clinical aspects. Angle Orthod 72:175–179; 180–184.

Segal GR, Schiffman PH, Tuncay OC 2004 Meta analysis of treatment-related factors of external apical root resorbtion. Orthod Craniofac Res 7:71–78.

Case 3

Summary

Lisa, an 18-year-old girl, had previous extraction of four first premolars and fixed appliance therapy to successfully correct her Class II division 1 malocclusion.

What do you notice in Figure 17.4?

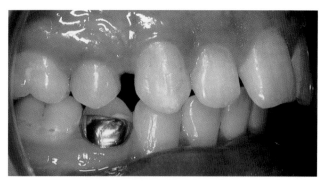

Fig. 17.4 Right buccal occlusion.

Lower arch aligned (note lingual retainer to $\overline{5|5}$ bands in place).

Space in $\underline{4|}$ area.

Increased overjet.

What does this indicate?

There has been relapse in the position of her teeth following treatment.

Why has this occurred?

The following factors are likely to destabilize the final orthodontic result.

Forces from the supporting tissues

Reorganization of principal periodontal ligament fibres and supporting alveolar bone occurs within 4–6 months after cessation of active tooth movmement. At least 7–8 months, however, is required for the supracrestal fibres to reorganize because of the slow turnover of the free gingival fibres. Rotational correction and space closure are, therefore, liable to relapse.

Forces from the orofacial soft tissues

Following appliance therapy, the teeth should be in a position of soft tissue balance. The original mandibular archform should remain unchanged as marked alteration in the inclination of the lower incisors will promote relapse. Limited proclination of the lower labial segment may be stable, however, in Class II Division 2 malocclusion, if the lower incisors were retroclined by a thumb-sucking habit or by a lower lip trap.

If a thumb- or digit-sucking habit is not ceased before treatment commences, its persistence will promote overjet relapse.

One third to one half of the labial surface of the upper incisors should be covered by the lower lip to give the best chance of stable overjet correction. Where the lips are grossly incompetent post-treatment, the upper incisor position will be inherently unstable and the mechanism by which an anterior oral seal is achieved will aggravate this further.

● Occlusal factors

A poor buccal segment interdigitation with displacing occlusal contacts and an unfavourable interincisal angulation will encourage instability.

● Post-treatment facial growth

Facial growth continues into adult life and, although of lesser magnitude than that observed during childhood, it varies among individuals. On average, females tend to demonstrate a backward mandibular rotation and this will not aid overjet stability. Late facial growth also impacts on the development of late lower incisor crowding.

● Retention regime

Firm rules do not exist for retention following active tooth movement but rather the retention regime should be decided individually for each case. A case-specific duration of retention is unknown at present. It is common practice, however, following fixed appliance therapy, to retain with removable retainers for a minimum of 3–6 months full-time followed by 6 months of night-only wear. It is acknowledged, however, that the only means of guaranteeing that tooth position is maintained unchanged long-term following completion of fixed appliance therapy is to advise long-term retention. Instead of a removable retainer, a bonded lingual retainer may be fitted to the lower incisors and canines; increasingly this is left in place permanently to prevent the development of late lower incisor crowding.

An inappropriate design of retainer, retention regime and/or inadequate compliance by the patient will facilitate relapse.

Key point

Relapse may be due to:
● Forces from:
    supporting tissues
    orofacial soft tissues
    occlusion
    facial growth.
● Inappropriate retainer design, retention regime and/or patient compliance.

What management options are there for this problem?

The following options exist:

1. Accept and monitor. Study models should record the current tooth position and occlusion, to allow comparison with the pre- and post-treatment study casts, and to act as a baseline from which to assess future occlusal change. If there is further relapse, then consider options 2 or 3 below.
2. Re-treatment. Full case assessment is required with appropriate radiographs and study models. Further upper arch extractions and fixed appliance therapy may be required for comprehensive recorrection of the malocclusion. Prolonged retention will be required thereafter.
3. A compromise plan would be to use an upper fixed appliance to retract the upper labial segment into the space that has opened in the first premolar extraction sites, accepting a slightly increased overjet. Then, prolonged retention would be required to maintain the result.

As Lisa is now a university student, she was not keen for further fixed appliance therapy and opted to accept and monitor the position of her teeth.

Recommended reading

Melrose C, Millett DT 1998 Toward a perspective on orthodontic retention? Am J Orthod Dentofacial Orthop 113:507–5142004.
Littlewood SJ, Millett DT, Doubleday B, Bearn DR, Worthington HV. Retention procedures for stabilizing tooth position after treatment with orthodontic braces (Cochrane Review). In: The Cochrane Library, Issue 1, 2004 John Wiley, Chichester.

For revision see Mind Map 17, page 163

18
Cleft lip and palate

Summary

Karen, a 9-year-old girl, is unhappy about the appearance of her teeth (**Fig. 18.1**). What is the cause and how will it be treated?

History

● Complaint

Karen does not like the crookedness and spacing of her upper front teeth. Her mother is aware that the bite of Karen's side teeth is not correct also and feels that she moves her jaw to the side when she closes her teeth together.

● History of complaint

Her baby front teeth were also crooked and spaced. Her mother has noticed the problem with Karen's bite for several months.

● Medical history

Karen was born with a cleft lip and palate, which has been repaired.

● Family history

There is no family history of cleft lip and palate.

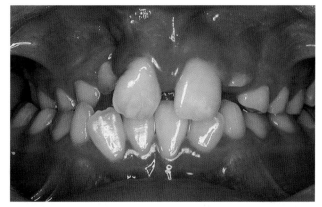

Fig. 18.1 Anterior occlusion at presentation.

What is the prevalence of cleft lip and palate?

It affects about 1 in 750 live births among Caucasians but the prevalence varies between racial groups as well as geographically, and is increasing. Cleft lip only is found in about 9% of all clefts whereas cleft of the lip and alveolus comprises about 3% of all clefts. Complete unilateral cleft lip and palate is the most common type of cleft and represents 50% of all clefts.

Is there a sex and side variation for cleft lip and palate?

Females are affected less frequently than males and the right side is involved less commonly than the left.

How does this malformation occur?

Failure of fusion of the median and lateral nasal processes and the maxillary process at about 4–6 weeks of intrauterine life leads to a cleft of the primary palate (the upper lip and the alveolus in the anterior region as far posteriorly as the incisive foramen). Cleft of the secondary palate (hard palate from incisive foramen back and soft palate) is due to failure of the palatal shelves to elevate and fuse at about 8 weeks.

Genetic and environmental factors, e.g. steroid therapy, folic acid deficiency or anticonvulsant drugs, interact in the aetiology.

> **Key point**
>
> Cleft lip and palate:
> - Prevalence 1 in 750 live Caucasian births.
> - Aetiology due to genetic and environmental factors.

Karen has been attending a Cleft Clinic at the Regional Dental Teaching Hospital since birth.

Why is this? What treatment will have been provided to date and what role have you to play as her general dental practitioner?

Due to the multidisciplinary care required, treatment is facilitated for the patient and family by coordinating management in a specialized centre by a team comprising an orthodontist, speech therapist and health visitor, as well as plastic, ENT and maxillofacial surgeons.

Treatment up until now is likely to have been as follows:

Neonatal period to 18 months: parental counselling by a member of the Cleft Lip and Palate Association and reassurance of the future treatment by an orthodontist and member of the surgical team.

Advice and support to the parents by a specialized health visitor, particularly in relation to feeding. In this case, feeding problems are likely to have been modest as the cleft only involves the primary palate.

Planning of lip closure: this usually occurs at 3 months. In this case closure of the alveolar defect may be undertaken at the same time. Where a palatal cleft exists, this is usually closed at 9–12 months.

● Primary dentition

First formal speech and hearing assessment at around 2 years and then speech therapy as required.

Regular speech and hearing assessments should be undertaken.

Consider lip revision at 4–5 years.

As a general dental practitioner your role is to:

Liaise with the Cleft Palate Team.

Provide dietary advice and oral hygiene instruction to the parents, at regular intervals, from eruption of the primary incisors.

Consider the use of fluoride tablets if the level of fluoride in the local domestic water supply is below 1 ppm.

Attend to any dental treatment required.

Your particular aim in dental care is to promote and maintain excellent dental health for Karen, thereby avoiding the need for restorative treatment or enforced loss of primary teeth through dental caries.

Key point

● Management of cleft lip and palate requires a team approach.

What skeletal/dental/occlusal problems are commonly found with cleft lip and palate?

Skeletally, there is a tendency for the maxilla and mandible to be retrognathic, the upper face height to be reduced and the lower face height to be increased. A Class III skeletal pattern is common.

On the cleft side, 2 is either absent, of abnormal size and/or shape, hypoplastic or as two conical teeth on either side of the cleft.

A supernumerary or supplemental tooth may exist on either side of the cleft.

1 is often rotated and tilted toward the cleft and may be hypoplastic.

Eruption is delayed.

Tooth size elsewhere in the mouth is small.

Class III incisor relationship is common with crossbite of one or both buccal segments and a lateral open bite.

Key point

● Incisor and buccal segment crossbites are common in repaired cleft lip and palate.

Examination
● Extraoral
What do you notice from Figure 18.2?

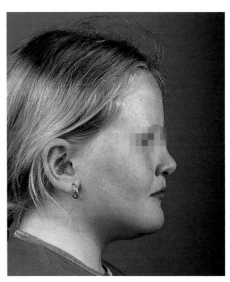

Fig. 18.2 a

Fig. 18.2 b

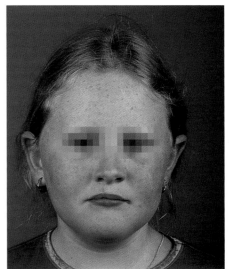

Fig. 18.2 (a) Profile. (b) Full face.

Karen has a Class I skeletal pattern with average FMPA and no obvious facial asymmetry. The lips are competent with a scar on the right side of the upper lip.

No clicks, locks or crepitus of the temporomandibular joints were detected.

How is lip closure achieved?

A Millard repair with or without its modifications is the most popular, aiming, after dissection, to place the lip muscles and alar base in their correct anatomical location. Whether subperiosteal or supraperiosteal dissection and skin-lengthening cuts are used to obtain tissue movement, remains controversial. The extent of alar cartilage dissection or the use of a vomer flap also remains unresolved.

● **Intraoral**

The appearance of the teeth is shown in Figures 18.1 and 18.3. What are your observations?

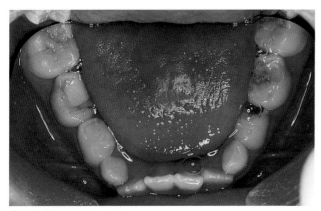

Fig. 18.3 a

Fig. 18.3 b

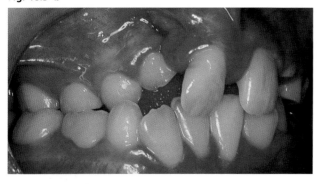

Fig. 18.3 c

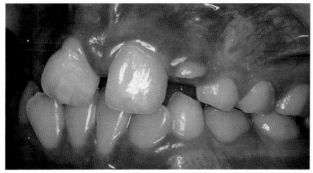

Fig. 18.3 (a) Lower occlusal view. (b) Right buccal occlusion. (c) Left buccal occlusion.

Oral hygiene is fair. Plaque deposits are visible on several teeth. The gingival appearance is consistent with mild marginal gingivitis.

$\dfrac{6\ e\ d\ c\ b\ 1\ |\ 1\ 2\ c\ d\ e\ 6}{6\ e\ d\ c\ 2\ 1\ |\ 1\ 2\ c\ d\ e\ 6}$ visible.

$\overline{e\ |\ e}$ restored; possible caries in $\overline{e\ |\ de}$; $\underline{1\ |}$ slightly hypoplastic.

Mild lower labial segment crowding.

Spaced upper labial segment with $\underline{1\ |}$ distolabially rotated.

The cleft repair involves the upper lip and alveolus—a bony depression is evident in the $\underline{2\ |}$ area.

Class II incisor relationship with average overbite; lower centreline shift to the right.

Right molar relationship half-unit Class II with buccal segment crossbite involving $\dfrac{6-c\ |}{6-c\ |}$; left molar relationship Class I.

In view of the unilateral crossbite of the right buccal segment, what should you check for? How would you do this?

It would be important to check if there is a mandibular displacement on the path of closure associated with the crossbite. As Karen's mother has already noticed a shift of the lower jaw on closure, a displacement is likely. To detect this, Karen should be instructed to maintain the tip of her tongue in contact with the back of her palate as she closes her teeth together. Careful observation should be made of first tooth contact on the path of closure and the extent and direction of any mandibular displacement into maximum intercuspation should be recorded.

There is a mandibular displacement to the right on closure resulting from premature contact of $\dfrac{c\ |}{c\ |}$.

Investigations
What investigations are required? Explain why

A dental panoramic tomogram should be taken to account for the presence and position of any unerupted teeth and to ascertain whether there are any permanent teeth absent.

An anterior maxillary occlusal radiograph is required to determine the extent of the alveolar cleft and the position of the permanent maxillary canine on the cleft side.

Karen's dental panoramic tomogram and standard occlusal radiograph are shown in Figure 18.4. What do you notice?

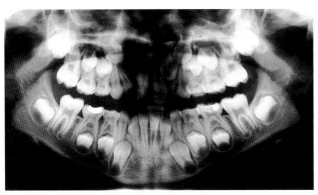

Fig. 18.4 a

Fig. 18.4 b

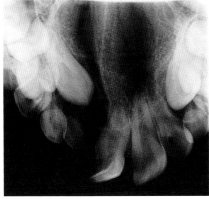

Fig. 18.4 (a) Dental panoramic tomogram. (b) Standard occlusal radiograph.

The dental panoramic tomogram shows:

Normal alveolar bone height except for the alveolar cleft in the $\underline{2|}$ area, which extends palatally to involve $\underline{3|}$.

- All permanent teeth are present except for $\underline{2|}$, $\overline{ed|de}$ are submerging.
- $\underline{1|}$ is hypoplastic; $\overline{e|e}$ appear to have secondary caries underneath the restorations with possible furcation radiolucencies.
- There is carious involvement of $\overline{d|d}$ distally.
- The anterior maxillary occlusal radiograph confirms the extent of the alveolar cleft, and when assessed in combination with the dental panoramic tomogram, it shows $\underline{3|}$ to be lying in the line of the arch.

Diagnosis
What is your diagnosis?

Generalized mild marginal gingivitis.
Repaired right unilateral cleft lip and alveolus.
Caries $\overline{ed|de}$.
Class III malocclusion on a Class I skeletal base with average FMPA.
Mandibular displacement to the right on closure on $\frac{c|}{c|}$.
Mild lower labial segment crowding.
Spaced upper labial segment with $\underline{1|}$ distolabially rotated; absent $\underline{2|}$.
Lower centreline to the right.
Right molar relationship half-unit Class II with buccal crossbite of the right buccal segments; left molar relationship Class I.

What is the IOTN DHC grade (see p. 183)?

5p due to cleft lip and palate.

Treatment
What are the aims of treatment at this stage?

Caries control.
Elimination of the mandibular displacement with correction of the right buccal segment crossbite.
Elimination of the alveolar cleft defect.

What would you do at this stage?

Reinforce oral hygiene practice in preparation for forthcoming orthodontic treatment.
Restore the lower primary molars.
Fissure seal the first permanent molars.
Liaise with the orthodontist on the cleft team regarding the planned orthodontic treatment.

What form do you envisage the orthodontic treatment to take?

Upper arch expansion, by a quadhelix appliance, to correct the buccal segment crossbite is likely to be underaken prior to alveolar bone grafting.

When is secondary alveolar bone grafting usually undertaken and what advantages does it confer?

It is usually undertaken between 8 and 11 years. It provides bone through which $\underline{3}$ can erupt, restores arch integrity, improves alar base support, aids closure of an oronasal fistula and allows orthodontic space closure.

The occlusion prior to bone grafting is shown in Figure 18.5. What may you consider at this stage?

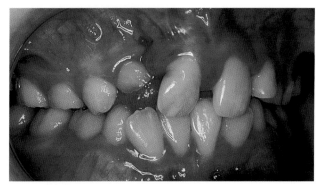

Fig. 18.5 Right buccal occlusion following crossbite correction with quadhelix.

Due to the advanced state of root resorption of c| it would be useful to remove this at least 3 weeks before grafting to allow time for socket healing, thereby improving the likelihood of graft success as an access route for oral infection is removed.

What treatment will be required following alveolar bone grafting?

Once 3 erupts, move the right upper buccal segment forward so 3 replaces 2.

Consider relief of crowding in the non-cleft quadrant and in the lower arch. Delay any lower arch extractions if orthognathic surgery is planned at a later date.

Fixed appliance therapy will be required for the active tooth movement described above.

Bonded retention will then be required to maintain upper labial segment alignment, and restorative treatment will be required to make 3 simulate an upper lateral incisor. In late teenage years consideration may be given to further lip revision or orthognathic surgery with rhinoplasty later, if a marked anteroposterior and/or vertical skeletal discrepancy exists.

In Karen's case, provided facial growth is reasonably favourable, orthognathic surgery may not be required.

Key point

Secondary alveolar bone grafting:
● Provides bone for 3 eruption.
● Restores arch integrity.
● Improves alar base support.
● Aids oronasal fistula closure.
● Allows orthodontic space closure.

Recommended reading

Bergland O, Semb G, Abyholm FE 1986 Elimination of the residual alveolar cleft by secondary bone grafting and subsequent orthodontic treatment. Cleft Palate J 23:175–205.

Rivkin CJ, Keith O, Crawford PJM, Hathorn IS 2000 Dental care for the patient with a cleft lip and palate. Part 1: From birth to the mixed dentition stage; Part 2: The mixed dentition stage through to adolescence and young adulthood. Br Dent J 118:78–83; 131–134.

Thom AR 1990 Modern management of the cleft lip and palate patient. Dent Update 17:402–408.

For revision see Mind Map 18, page 164

19

Nursing and early childhood caries

Summary

Kelly-Ann is only 3. She has been brought to the dentist by her mother because her upper front teeth are 'wearing away' (**Fig. 19.1**). What has caused this and how may it be treated?

History

The teeth apparently never came through properly and were never white like the rest of her teeth. There has been no pain from the teeth and Kelly-Ann is eating and drinking normally.

Medical history

Kelly-Ann is a healthy infant. She has had all her vaccinations and has had no illnesses. She has never been on any medication.

Examination

Extraorally there is no swelling and no facial asymmetry. Intraorally she is in the full primary dentition with the second primary molars having just erupted. There is caries affecting the upper incisors and all first primary molars.

What is the cause of this pattern of decay?

'Nursing caries', or 'nursing bottle mouth' or 'bottle mouth caries'.

What can cause this?

Consumption of a sweetened drink or fruit-flavoured drink from a bottle or dinky feeder, especially if the

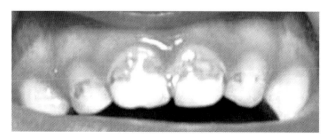

Fig. 19.1 Early cavitation in nursing caries.

feeder is constantly in the mouth or the child falls asleep with it in the mouth.

Persistent on-demand breast feeding at night after 12 months of age (child is allowed to sleep on the breast) may cause caries in exceptional circumstances. There are many biological and social variables that confound this complex relationship.

As can be seen, the term 'nursing caries' is probably the most accurate as it encompasses both breast feeding and bottle feeding.

Why are the teeth affected in this pattern?

Teeth become carious in the order in which they erupt with the exception of the lower primary incisors, which are protected by two major mechanisms: the position of the submandibular ducts that open adjacent to these teeth; the position of the tongue in suckling, which covers the lower incisors (**Fig. 19.2**).

What additional factors make the upper primary incisors more predisposed to caries?

High bow-shaped upper lip in infants that does not cover the upper incisors and results in an increased evaporation of any saliva on these teeth.

Gravity, which keeps submandibular saliva pooled around the lower incisors and less likely to reach the upper incisors.

Any liquid with sugar that is allowed to bathe the teeth on a frequent basis will cause caries. This is especially so at night when the protective function of saliva reduces as less saliva is produced. Even breast milk, formula milk or cows' milk with their lowered natural sugars can still be cariogenic on this basis.

> ### Key point
>
> Nursing caries:
> - Affects teeth in order of eruption.
> - Lower incisors are protected by saliva.
> - Can be caused by any sugar-containing liquid.

What should be your advice about night-time feeding?

Only water should be given during the night after 12 months of age.

The term early childhood caries (ECC) is an additional term used to describe any caries presenting in the primary dentition of young children. Some children present with extensive caries that does not follow the 'nursing caries' pattern and have multiple carious teeth, and may be slightly older at 3, 4 or 5 years of age at initial presentation.

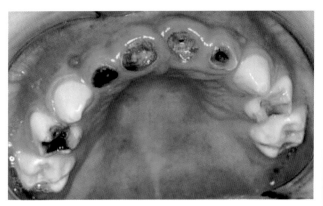

Fig. 19.2 Classical distribution of affected teeth in nursing caries in upper arch.

How could you identify preschool children in need of dental care?

Encourage parents to bring their children for a dental check-up as soon as the child has teeth.

Make contact with local health visitors, baby clinics, and mother and baby groups via the local general medical practice.

Treatment

Kelly-Ann is in a high risk for caries group. List all the main factors you can think of for placing someone in the high risk group for dental caries? See **Table 19.1**.

Table 19.1 'High risk' factors for caries	
Risk factor	**Aetiology**
Clinical evidence	New lesions
	Premature extractions
	Anterior caries or restorations
	Multiple restorations
	No fissure sealants
	Fixed appliance orthodontics
	Partial dentures
Dietary habits	Frequent sugar intake
Social history	Social deprivation
	High caries in siblings
	Low knowledge of dental disease
	Irregular attendance
	Ready availability of snacks
	Low dental aspirations
Use of fluoride	Drinking water not fluoridated
	No fluoride supplements
	No fluoride toothpaste
Plaque control	Infrequent, ineffective cleaning
	Poor manual control
Saliva	Low flow rate
	Low buffering capacity
	High *Streptococcus mutans* and *Lactobacillus* counts
Medical history	Medically compromised
	Physical disability
	Intellectual disability
	Xerostomia
	Long-term cariogenic medicine

What fluoride regime would you suggest to her mother?

Fluoride paste. As a high risk subject, consideration should be given to a 1000 or 1450 ppm fluoride paste rather than 450–600 ppm children's paste.

Fluoride supplements. These should be considered in high risk of caries subjects and in children in whom dental disease would pose a serious risk to general health (e.g. risk of infectious endocarditis). Such supplementation is only effective if given long term and regularly.

What information is essential before prescribing fluoride supplements?

The amount of fluoride in the local water. Telephone the local water supplier for this information.

What is the currently recommended fluoride supplementation regime in the UK (see Table 19.2)?

● Professionally applied fluorides

Site-specific application of fluoride varnish can be very valuable in the management of early, smooth surface and approximal carious lesions. Recent evidence suggests that passage of floss through a contact point between primary molars by parents can greatly enhance prevention and early treatment of approximal lesions. The most commonly used varnish—5% sodium fluoride—has 22 600 ppm and should be applied very sparingly to specific areas three times a year.

Why can Kelly-Ann not have fluoride mouthwash?

These are contraindicated in children less than 6 years of age because more than half the mouthwash will be swallowed.

What other forms of preventive care does she need?

● Toothbrushing instruction

Preschool children need help from their parents if effective oral hygiene is to be maintained. Brushing needs to start as soon as the first tooth erupts. Standing or kneeling behind the child in front of a sink or mirror is often the best way to brush a young child's teeth. Supervision of brushing is important so that an appro-

Table 19.2 Recommended dosage schedule for fluoride supplements in areas where the water supply contains less than 0.3 ppm fluoride	
Age	**mg fluoride per day**
6 months to 3 years	0.25 mg
3–6 years	0.50 mg
6 years	1.00 mg

priate amount of paste is placed on the brush to prevent/reduce ingestion of paste. Teeth should be cleaned at least once a day.

● Diet analysis

The only way to effectively do this is by a 3- or 4-day written analysis. It is important to try and obtain 1 day's history from a weekend as they are invariably different from weekdays. In modern society it is common for most parents to work and the child to be looked after by a carer or nursery. It is critical to establish who is the carer during weekdays and weekends. Advice needs to be clear at all times, but if it has to be relayed from a parent in the surgery to a carer then it needs to be clear, succinct and written. Frequent consumption of sugar-containing drinks and feeds is the key aetiological feature in many children with preschool caries. Reducing the frequency of sugar-containing snacks is the key message. If the child is a 'poor eater' there is need to build up the amount of food at mealtimes and, therefore, reduce the need for frequent snacking. Children do not need lots of fizzy drinks or fruit-based drinks. They often take them to make up for calories missed at mealtimes. Only milk and water should be taken between meals. A small amount of fruit-based drink can more safely be taken with a meal. As mentioned above, it is critical to stop the night-time bottle.

In your dietary advice you must be *practical*, *personal* and *positive*. Try to avoid making the parent feel excessively guilty but concentrate on practical strategies. It is probably unreasonable to give out more than four pieces of written advice. These should concentrate on daytime drinks, night-time drinks, between-meal snacks, and making sure the child has no food or drink for 1 hour before going to bed and then cleans the teeth just before bed.

Kelly-Ann has the early cavitation on her upper incisors that you see in Figure 19.1. She also has early cavitated occlusal caries in her first primary molars.

How would you restore the upper incisors?

These can be restored with a compomer, which has a good bond strength to enamel and dentine. Compomers have good mechanical properties and in this situation will be as durable as composite.

How would you restore the cavitated first primary molars?

Compomer similarly will be the restorative material of choice.

All this work, because it is not extensive, could probably be achieved with a slow handpiece and excavator. However, if Kelly-Ann is apprehensive of the 'drill' then an alternative way of caries removal will have to be found.

What recently developed method of caries removal, without a handpiece, may be applicable here?

Carisolv, which accomplishes caries removal by chemo-mechanical means. Carisolv consists of a pink gel that contains mainly the amino acids leucine, lysine and glutamic acid, and hypochlorite. In addition there is cellulose and a colouring agent, erythrocin. The amino acids and hypochlorite work to separate carious dentine from sound dentine and the carious dentine is removed with the aid of special hand instruments that have different cutting edges and hand actions to excavators. They are used in a whisking, rotating, or up and down movement. Because the sound dentine is not stimulated by the temperature or vibration of a handpiece, or the temperature changes of a 3 in 1 spray, it is a painless procedure. The cavity should be dried by saline-dampened cotton wool, then dry cotton wool, prior to restoring with an adhesive material. Bond strengths to adhesive materials are the same as conventionally prepared cavities.

How is pain relief best achieved in the child with nursing caries in Figure 19.2?

This is a case where general anaesthesia for teeth removal is justified. This is covered in Chapter 22.

Recommended reading

Ripa LW 1988 Nursing caries: a comprehensive review. Paediatr Dent 10:268–282.

For revision see Mind Map 19, page 165

20

The uncooperative child

Summary

Liam is 5. He is shaking and tearful as he is brought into the surgery. His mother says he has been in pain from his teeth for a long time (**Fig. 20.1**). How would you manage Liam and his dental treatment?

What do you understand by the term behaviour management?

Based on scientific principles, the proper implementation of behaviour management requires an understanding of these principles. It requires skills in empathy, communication, coaching and listening.

The goals are to establish communication, alleviate fear and anxiety, deliver quality dental care, build a trusting relationship between dentist and child, and promote the child's positive attitude towards oral/dental health.

All decisions must be based on a benefit versus risk evaluation. Parents/legal guardians share in the decision-making process regarding treatment of their children.

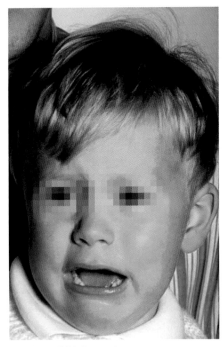

Fig. 20.1 In pain and frightened.

What history is important in Liam's case?

Liam's dental history. It is crucial to identify any previous episodes either at the dentist, doctor, or hospital, usually involving needles, that may have frightened him. If there are no previous precipitating factors he may have been frightened by stories or comments from his peers or family.

Family dental history. Parental fear, and a negative attitude toward dental and oral health, can significantly affect the cooperation of a child.

Liam's development. Delayed development and poor cognition can affect the ability of a child to understand what you are trying to do to help. Children with a negative image of themselves who have never succeeded well at anything will be more difficult to treat. They often give up because they 'never succeed' and are often called 'failures' by their parents or peers.

Communicative management is the most fundamental form of behaviour management. It is the basis for establishing a relationship with a child that will allow you to successfully complete dental procedures and help the child develop a positive attitude toward dental health.

What main forms of communicative management are there?

Voice control.
Non-verbal communication.
Tell–show–do.
Positive reinforcement.
Distraction.
Parental presence/absence.

● Voice control

Description: Voice control is a controlled alteration of voice volume, tone or pace to influence and direct the patient's behaviour.

Objectives:
1. To gain the patient's attention and compliance.
2. To avert negative or avoidance behaviour.
3. To establish appropriate adult–child roles.

Indications: May be used with any patient.

Contraindications: None.

● Non-verbal communication

Description: Non-verbal communication is the reinforcement and guidance of behaviour through appropriate contact, posture and facial expression.

Objectives:
1. To enhance the effectiveness of other communicative management techniques.
2. To gain or maintain the patient's attention and compliance.

Indications: May be used with any patient.

Contraindications: None.

Tell–show–do

Description: Tell–show–do is a technique of behaviour shaping used by many paediatric professionals. The technique involves verbal explanations of procedures in phrases appropriate to the developmental level of the patient (Tell); demonstrations for the patient of the visual, auditory, olofactory and tactile aspects of the procedure in a carefully defined, non-threatening setting (Show); and then, without deviating from the explanation and demonstration, completion of the procedure (Do). The tell–show–do technique is used with communication skills (verbal and non-verbal) and positive reinforcement.

Objectives:
1. To teach the patient important aspects of the dental visit and familiarize the patient with the dental setting.
2. To shape the patient's response to procedures through desensitization and well-described expectations.

Indications: May be used with any patient.
Contraindications: None.

Positive reinforcement

Description: In the process of establishing desirable patient behaviour, it is essential to give appropriate feedback. Positive reinforcement is an effective technique to reward desired behaviours and thus strengthen the recurrence of those behaviours. Social reinforcers include positive voice modulation, facial expression, verbal praise and appropriate physical demonstrations of affection by all members of the dental team. Non-social reinforcers include tokens and toys.

Objective:
1. To reinforce desired behaviour.

Indications: May be useful for any patient.
Contraindications: None.

Distraction

Description: Distraction is the technique of diverting the patient's attention from what may be perceived as an unpleasant procedure.

Objectives:
1. To decrease the perception of unpleasantness.
2. To avert negative or avoidance behaviour.

Indications: May be used with any patient.
Contraindications: None.

Parental presence/absence

Description: This technique involves using the presence or absence of the parent to gain cooperation for treatment. A wide diversity exists in practitioner philosophy and parental attitude regarding parents' presence or absence during paediatric dental treatment. Practitioners are united in the fact that communication between dentist and child is paramount and that this communication demands focus on the part of both parties. Children's responses to their parents' presence or absence can range from very beneficial to very detrimental. It is the responsibility of practitioners to determine the communication methods that best optimize the treatment setting; recognizing their own skills, the abilities of the particular child and the desires of the specific parent involved.

Objectives:
1. To gain the patient's attention and compliance.
2. To avert negative or avoidance behaviours.
3. To establish appropriate adult–child roles.
4. To enhance the communication environment.

Indications: May be used with any patient.
Contraindications: None.

All these communication techniques integrate to enhance the evolution of a compliant and relaxed patient. It is an ongoing subjective process rather than a singular technique and is often the extension of the personality of the dentist.

Key point

The objectives of distraction are:
- To decrease the perception of unpleasantness.
- To avert negative or avoidance behaviour.

Examination

After spending some time talking to Liam and showing him that you are genuine in wanting to help, he allows you to look at his teeth. There are two carious first primary molars in the mandible. All the other teeth are sound. Liam has been frightened by stories from his friends. His family are very supportive and are regular attenders.

Liam responds well to communicative management but, although he wants to have his treatment done he just cannot override his fear of the unknown.

What additional help might you consider giving Liam?

Sedation—there are two options for sedation, either oral or inhalational sedation.

Oral sedation is now an increasingly viable option using midazolam. A number of recent studies have shown that its use in a dose of 0.3–0.5 mg/kg, depending on age, has been therapeutically effective in producing effective sedation that has allowed subsequent dental treatment. The objectives, indications and contraindications for it are:

Objectives:
1. To reduce or eliminate anxiety.
2. To reduce untoward movement and reaction to dental treatment.
3. To enhance communication and patient cooperation.

4. To increase tolerance for longer appointments.
5. To aid in treatment of the mentally, physically or medically compromised patient.
6. To raise the patient's pain threshold.

Indications:

1. Fearful, anxious patients in whom basic behaviour management has not been successful.
2. Patients who cannot cooperate due to a lack of psychological or emotional maturity and/or mental, physical or medical disability.
3. Patients for whom the use of sedation may protect the developing psyche and/or reduce medical risk.

Contraindications:

1. The cooperative patient with minimal dental needs.
2. Predisposing medical conditions that would make sedation inadvisable.

Inhalational sedation has been known to be an effective and safe method of reducing anxiety and enhancing effective communication for the last 25 years. Its onset of action is rapid, the depth of sedation is easily titrated and reversible, and recovery is rapid and complete. Additionally, nitrous oxide mediates a variable degree of analgesia, amnesia and gag reflex reduction.

The need to diagnose and treat, as well as the safety of the patient and practitioner, should be considered before the use of nitrous oxide. The decision to use nitrous oxide must take into consideration:

1. Alternative behaviour management modalities.
2. Dental needs of the patient.
3. The effect on the quality of dental care.
4. The patient's emotional development.
5. The patient's physical considerations.

Written informed consent must be obtained from a legal guardian and documented in the patient's record prior to use of nitrous oxide.

The patient's record should include:

1. Informed consent.
2. Indication for use.
3. Nitrous oxide dosage:
   (a) Percent nitrous oxide/oxygen and/or flow rate.
   (b) Duration of the procedure.
   (c) Post-treatment oxgenation procedure.

Objectives:

1. To reduce or eliminate anxiety.
2. To reduce untoward movement and reaction to dental treatment.
3. To enhance communication and patient cooperation.
4. To raise the pain reaction threshold.
5. To increase tolerance for longer appointments.
6. To aid in treatment of the mentally/physically disabled, or medically compromised patient.
7. To reduce gagging.

Indications:

1. A fearful, anxious or obstreperous patient.
2. Certain mentally, physically or medically compromised patients.

3. A patient whose gag reflex interferes with dental care.
4. A patient for whom profound local anaesthesia cannot be obtained.

Contraindications:

1. May be contraindicated in some chronic obstructive pulmonary diseases.
2. May be contraindicated in certain patients with severe emotional disturbances or drug-related dependencies.
3. Patients in the first trimester of pregnancy.
4. May be contraindicated in patients with sickle cell disease.
5. Patients treated with bleomycin sulfate.

Liam had inhalational sedation, which enabled him to complete his treatment and overcome his fear of local anaesthesia. Unfortunately, there are some children for whom inhalational sedation will not work and general anaesthesia (GA) is the only option that will allow relief of pain and completion of dental treatment.

Key point

The patient's record in inhalational sedation should include:
● Informed consent.
● Indications for use.
● Nitrous oxide dosage.

What are the indications for general anaesthesia?

Patients who are unable to cooperate due to a lack of psychological or emotional maturity, and/or mental, physical or medical disability.

Patients for whom local anaesthesia is ineffective because of acute infection, anatomic variations or allergy.

The extremely uncooperative, fearful, anxious or uncommunicative child or adolescent.

Patients requiring significant surgical procedures.

Patients for whom the use of general anaesthesia may protect the developing psyche and/or reduce medical risks.

Patients requiring immediate, comprehensive oral/dental care.

What are the contraindications for general anaesthesia?

A healthy, cooperative patient with minimal dental need.

Predisposing medical conditions that would make GA inadvisable.

General anaesthesia is a controlled state of unconsciousness accompanied by a loss of protective reflexes, including the ability to maintain an airway independently and respond purposefully to physical stimulation or verbal command. It should only be provided in premises with resuscitation capability and intensive care back-up. All equipment must follow current guidelines.

Parental or legal guardian informed consent must be obtained and documented prior to the use of general anaesthesia. The patient's record should include:

Informed consent.

Indications for the use of GA.

● Informed consent

Regardless of the behaviour management techniques utilized by the individual practitioner, all management decisions must be based on a subjective evaluation weighing benefit and risk to the child. Considerations regarding need of treatment, consequences of deferred treatment and potential physical/emotional trauma must be entered into the decision-making equation.

Delivery of dental treatment is often a complex decision. Decisions regarding the use of behaviour management techniques other than communicative management cannot be made solely by the dentist. Decisions must involve a legal guardian and, if appropriate, the child. The dentist serves as the expert about dental care, i.e. the need for treatment and the techniques by which treatment can be delivered. The legal guardian shares with the practitioner the decision whether to treat or not treat and must be consulted regarding treatment strategies and potential risks. Therefore, the successful completion of diagnostic and therapeutic services is viewed as a partnership of dentist, legal guardian and child.

Although the behaviour management techniques included in this chapter are used frequently, parents may not be entirely familiar with them. It is important that the dentist inform the legal guardian about the nature of the technique to be used, its risks, benefits and any alternative techniques. All questions must be answered. This is the essence of informed consent.

Recommended reading

Guidelines for behavior management 1999 American Academy of Pediatric Dentistry reference manual 1999–2000. Paediatr Dent 21:42–46.

Hosey MT 2002 Managing anxious children: the use of conscious sedation in paediatric dentistry. UK National Clinical Guideline. Int J Paed Dent 12:359–372.

Pinkham JR 1995 Personality development. Managing behaviour of the cooperative pre-school child. Dent Clin North Am 39:771–787.

For revision see Mind Map 20, page 166

21

Disorders of eruption and exfoliation

Case 1
Summary
Beth was only 20 days old when it was noticed she had two teeth at the front of the lower jaw (**Fig. 21.1**).

What is the correct terminology for these early erupting teeth?
If the teeth are present at birth then 'natal' is the correct term. If they are not present at birth but erupt within the first month of life then 'neonatal' is correct.

The prevalence rates for both natal and neonatal teeth are reported as 1 in 2000–3000 live births. The most commonly presenting tooth is the lower central incisor. More rarely, maxillary incisors or first molars have been reported. The early eruption is thought to be caused by the ectopic position of the tooth germ during fetal life. Natal and neonatal teeth may follow a sporadic pattern or they may be familial. However, they can be associated with specific syndromes:

Pachyonychia congenita.
Ellis–van Creveld.
Hallermann–Strieff.

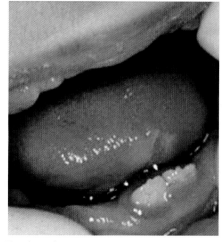

Fig. 21.1 Natal teeth.

What are the main problems associated with natal and neonatal teeth?
Mobility.
Ulceration of ventral surface of tongue.
Nipple soreness (breast-feeding mothers).

The teeth are mobile because the development of the tooth is consistent with age. Only about five-sixths of the crown is formed and not normally any root. Additionally, the crown is occasionally dilacerated and the enamel hypoplastic or hypomineralized.

Excessive mobility is a danger to the airway from aspiration and the tooth should be removed. Care should be taken to ensure that the entire tooth including the pulpal tissue is removed, otherwise dentine and a root will form, which will require eventual removal. If teeth can be left then continued root development will occur.

Nipple soreness may occasionally necessitate tooth removal.

Ulceration on the ventral surface of the tongue may respond to carmellose sodium oral paste. Smoothing of the incisal edges with soflex discs may also help.

What factors can cause generalized premature eruption but still be considered as 'normal'?
Familial—a family history is a common finding.
Children with high birth weights.
Race—generally Negroids tend to erupt their permanent teeth earlier than Mongoloids, who are in turn in advance of Caucasians. Racial group does not seem to affect eruption times of primary teeth but eruption patterns can vary in the primary dentition.
Sex—females tend to erupt permanent teeth several months ahead of males.

The opposite of premature eruption is delayed eruption.

When is generalized delay in eruption of primary teeth expected?
Preterm infants.
Very low birth weight infants.

What conditions may lead to a generalized retarded eruption of teeth in both primary and permanent dentitions?
Chromosomal abnormalities—Down and Turner syndromes.
Gross nutritional deficiency.
Hypothyroidism/hypopituitarism.
Hereditary gingival fibromatosis (HGF).
Acquired gingival overgrowth (drug-induced).

What specific condition is associated with grossly delayed or failed eruption of teeth in the permanent dentition?
Cleidocranial dysplasia. This is an autosomal dominantly inherited condition where, in addition to multiple super-

numerary teeth causing delayed exfoliation of primary teeth and delayed eruption of permanent teeth, there is aplasia of commonly the distal end or total absence of the clavicles.

What local factors can account for delayed eruption of permanent teeth?

Supernumerary teeth or odontomes.
Ectopic crypt positions of permanent teeth.
Cystic change in the follicle of permanent teeth.
Crowding.
Thickened mucosa due to early primary tooth removal.

Key point

Natal and neonatal teeth may need to be removed if:
- Mobility causes concern about inhalation.
- Ulceration under the ventral surface of the tongue persists.
- Nipple soreness is significant.

Exfoliation of teeth (like eruption) can be either premature or delayed.

Case 2
Summary

George was 3 years of age when his mother first noticed that his lower primary incisors were loose.

History

George was born after a normal pregnancy and delivery but had problems after birth with recurrent coughs and colds, upper and lower respiratory tract infections, and oral ulceration. He was extensively investigated and was confirmed as having a cyclical neutropenia.

● Dental history

George and his mother had regular toothbrush instruction and his oral hygiene was excellent. He also used 0.2% chlorhexidine gel at night instead of fluoridated toothpaste. Despite these efforts he exfoliated his lower primary incisors between age 4 and 5 and by his sixth birthday he had erupted his lower permanent central incisors and first permanent molars (**Figs 21.2a** and **b**).

Premature loss of primary teeth is an important diagnostic event, as most conditions causing it are potentially serious and warrant immediate investigation (**Box 21.1**).

Generally teeth may be lost early because of:
Metabolic disturbances
Severe periodontal disease
Loss of alveolar bone support
Self-injury or non-accidental injury
George will continue to have regular dental care and

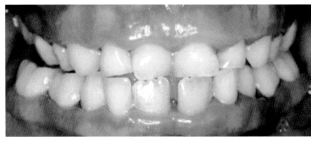

Fig. 21.2 a

Fig. 21.2 b

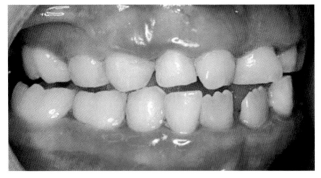

Fig. 21.2 (a,b) Cyclical neutropenia.

supervision of brushing. Even in the presence of immaculate plaque control we can expect that his neutrophil defect will predispose him to periodontal disease and premature loss of some if not all his permanent teeth.

The opposite of premature exfoliation is delayed exfoliation.

What causes delayed exfoliation of primary teeth?

Double primary teeth.
Hypodontia affecting permanent successors.
Ectopically placed permanent successors.

Box 21.1 Differential diagnosis of causes of premature exfoliation of primary and permanent teeth

Neutropenias and qualitative neutrophil defects:
    Cyclical neutropenia
    Congenital neutropenia (Kostmann's disease)
    Prepubertal periodontitis
    Juvenile periodontitis
    Leucocyte adhesion defect
    Papillon–Lefèvre syndrome
    Chediak–Higashi disease
Langerhans cell histiocytosis—leading to bony destruction
Hypophosphatasia with aplasia or hypoplasia of cementum
Self-injury in either a psychotic disorder or the congenital insensitivity to pain syndrome
Ehlers–Danlos syndrome (Type VIII)—disorder of collagen formation causing progressive periodontal destruction
Scurvy—loss of tooth due to failure of proline hydroxylation and collagen synthesis

---

Trauma or periradicular infection of primary teeth causing interruption of physiological resorption.
Infraocclusion or ankylosis.

Double primary teeth are associated in 40% of cases with an abnormality of number of the permanent dentition. Parents should be advised of this and a dental panoramic tomogram should be taken around the age of 6.

Infraocclusion is the preferred term for either 'sub-merged teeth' or 'ankylosis' when describing teeth that have failed to achieve or maintain their occlusal relationship to adjacent or opposing teeth. Most commonly, primary teeth have reached a normal occlusal level before becoming infraoccluded. Rarely there may be primary failure of eruption of primary and permanent teeth in the same quadrant in the same person.

The tooth most commonly affected is the mandibular first primary molar. Males and females are affected equally. Infraoccluded primary teeth are associated with a higher incidence of absent permanent successors.

Key point

Infraocclusion:
- Mandibular first primary molar most commonly affected.
- More common in primary teeth than in permanent teeth.
- Equal sex ratio.
- Higher incidence of absent permanent successors.

How is infraocclusion graded?

Grade I	Occlusal level above contact point of adjacent tooth.
Grade II	Occlusal level at contact point of adjacent tooth.
Grade III	Occlusal level below contact point of adjacent tooth.

Grade III infraocclusions, if progressive, may be completely reincluded by the surrounding hard and soft tissues.

Radiographs of infraoccluded teeth show blurring or absence of the periodontal space.

● Treatment options in infraocclusion

These are considered in Chapter 6.

Recommended reading

Winter GB 2001 Anomalies of tooth formation and eruption. In: Welbury RR (ed) Paediatric dentistry, 2nd edn. Oxford University Press, Oxford, pp 271–298.

For revision see Mind Map 21, page 167

22
Pain control and carious teeth

Summary

Paul is 5 years old. He is in pain from one of his upper back teeth. He has never had any treatment before. How would you manage Paul's problem?

What questions do you need to ask regarding the pain?

Site—ask him to point to the tooth.

Severity—does the pain stop him from playing or sleeping?

Onset—what causes it. Is it in response to hot, cold or sweet stimuli, or does it occur spontaneously? Does it wake him up from sleep?

Character—is it a sharp pain or is it dull and throbbing?

Duration—how long does it last?

The characteristics of the pain of reversible and irreversible pulpitis are shown in **Table 22.1**.

Table 22.1 Pain characteristics

Reversible	Irreversible
Transient or short duration (minutes)	Long duration
Response to hot, cold, sweet	Response to pressure (chewing)
	Spontaneous
Sharp	Throbbing
Doesn't stop play or sleep	Stops play or sleep

The initial management of a child attending in pain is often constrained by possible lack of sleep on behalf of the child or time available to the dentist to treat this extra 'emergency patient'.

What dressings can help manage pulpitis initially?

After gentle excavation of the softest layer of coronal caries:

Zinc oxide eugenol cement (e.g. Kalzinol or Intermediate Restorative Material—IRM).

Polyantibiotic and steroid pastes (e.g. Ledermix) placed underneath zinc oxide eugenol cements or glass ionomer cement (GIC).

Formocresol 1 : 5 dilution on cotton pledget, covered by a suitable cement dressing, can be useful with an exposure or near exposure of the pulp.

If a tooth is abscessed then there is often significant coronal destruction. The pulp chamber of such teeth can often be accessed by gentle excavation, and then a dressing of 1 : 5 dilution formocresol on some cotton wool placed within the chamber and sealed with cement will often lead to resolution of the swelling.

An acute and/or spreading infection or swelling may require the prescription of antibiotics. This is discussed in Chapter 24. Antibiotics should only be prescribed for pain in the absence of swelling for immunosuppressed patients. Analgesics may be necessary for pain (**Table 22.2**).

Table 22.2 Dosages for common paediatric analgesics

Drug	Dosage
Paracetamol	20 mg/kg initially then 15 mg/kg every 4 hours Maximum 24-hour dosage 90 mg/kg Ensure adequate hydration
Ibuprofen (NSAID)	5–10 mg/kg every 8 hours Can be used in conjunction with paracetamol Best given with food and drink.

Dressing open cavities has a number of advantages:

Simple introduction to dental procedures.

Oral mutans streptococci count is reduced when excavation of gross caries is accomplished. If the cavity is then completely sealed by a GIC there is evidence that the viability of the remaining organisms reduce and caries progression is greatly reduced. This buys the dentist time to institute preventive and behaviour management programmes before reassessing teeth with temporary restorations.

GIC cements act as a fluoride reservoir.

Makes toothbrushing and eating more comfortable.

History

Questioning suggested a reversible pulpitis in the upper left quadrant but with recent features of an irreversible nature.

Examination

Paul has no extraoral swelling or asymmetry. Intraorally he has all his primary teeth with the exception of $\overline{a|}$ and $\overline{|a}$, which have just exfoliated. $\overline{1|}$ and $\overline{|1}$ are just erupting. There is mesial occlusal caries with loss of the marginal ridge on $d|$. The $|e$ is grossly carious (**Fig. 22.1**). There are no associated soft tissue swellings.

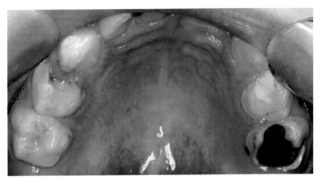

Fig. 22.1 Caries affecting d| and |e .

What investigation is essential to allow you to formulate a treatment plan?

Bitewing radiographs are necessary to diagnose approximal caries in primary molars with their wide contact areas. Radiographs will increase the diagnosed yield of caries by 50%. Frequency of subsequent bitewing radiographs will depend on the classification of caries risk: high should have radiographs 6–12 monthly; medium 12–18 monthly; low 18–24 monthly. In Paul's case a small amount of occlusal caries was confirmed in e| .

Key point

Advantages of dressing open cavities are:
- Introduction to dental procedures.
- Reduction of *Streptococcus mutans* count.
- GIC acts as a fluoride reservoir.
- Eating and toothbrushing are more comfortable.

Treatment

Initial temporization of d| and |e was with Ledermix paste under IRM cement. A preventive and behaviour management programme was started. e| was restored with an adhesive restoration.

What is your definitive treatment plan for d| and |e ?

Both these teeth require primary molar pulp treatment. Although d| is less affected by caries it has lost its mesial marginal ridge and will have histological evidence of inflammation in the coronal pulp.

What types of primary molar pulp treatment are there?

Vital pulpotomy. Coronal pulp is removed under local anaesthesia (LA) and the pulp stumps dressed for 5 minutes with 1 : 5 dilution formocresol. The chamber is then filled with zinc oxide eugenol cement.

Non-vital pulpotomy. This is a two-stage procedure and is used when there is non-vital tissue in the root canals or signs of soft tissue infection. A pledget of cotton wool with 1 : 5 dilution of formocresol is sealed into the chamber for 1–4 weeks with temporary cement. At the second appointment, if symptoms and signs have gone, then the tooth is restored with zinc oxide eugenol as above.

Devitalizing pulpotomy. This is a two-stage procedure that is used when anaesthesia cannot be gained. A pledget of devitalizing paste containing local anaesthetic and paraformaldehyde is sealed into the cavity/chamber with temporary cement for 1–4 weeks. At the second visit the coronal pulp can be removed without LA and restored as in vital pulpotomy.

Pulpectomy. This is also used when there is non-vital tissue in the root canals. The canals are instrumented with files and the canals filled with zinc oxide cement on a spiral filler.

The decision regarding which type of pulpotomy is applicable can only be made once treatment starts and clinical findings are taken into account. Pulp treatment should, ideally, always be completed under LA (with exception of devitalizing pulpotomy where LA either has not worked or cannot be given for behavioural reasons).

What is the appropriate restorative material after pulp treatment?

The techniques employed for definitive restorations in young children should take into account the active nature of the disease in the young child. The use of adhesive restorations should be limited to occlusal and small approximal cavities. Extensive cavities, teeth with two or more carious surfaces, and teeth after pulpotomy or pulpectomy should be restored with stainless steel crowns. Amalgam is still widely used as a restorative material but adhesive materials, especially polyacid-modified resins (compomers), and composite resins may be preferred as they have been shown to be as durable if they are placed under appropriate conditions with adequate isolation. Cermet cements are not appropriate restorations for primary teeth.

Extraction of teeth will be required if they are unrestorable or if there is acute pain and infection (Chapter 23). In preschool children the extraction of one or two teeth may be able to be accomplished under LA with oral or inhalation sedation. However, if extractions are required in two or more quadrants then a GA carried out in an appropriate setting is the treatment of choice. In these cases where GA is employed in young children the treatment planning should be radical and should aim to prevent a repeat GA in the future.

When planning extractions it is important to consider the need for balancing extractions. Factors such as the likelihood of continued future attendance and cooperation of the child should also be borne in mind. In preschool children with extensive caries, extraction of first primary molars with maintenance and restoration of second primary molars where possible is often a good plan. This limits the risk of further decay by eliminating posterior teeth interproximal contact areas.

Key point

The main types of primary molar pulp treatment are:
- Vital pulpotomy.
- Non-vital pulpotomy.
- Devitalization pulpotomy.
- Pulpectomy.

Recommended reading

Cameron A, Widmer R (eds) 2003 Pain control for children. In: Handbook of pediatric dentistry, 2nd edn. St Louis, Mosby-Wolfe, pp 19–21.
Fayle SA 2001 Treatment of dental caries in the pre-school child. In: Welbury RR (ed) Paediatric dentistry, 2nd edn. Oxford University Press, Oxford, pp 115–132.

For revision see Mind Map 22, page 168

23

Facial swelling and dental abscess

Summary

Peter is 12. He attended with a large facial swelling after an episode of trauma 3 weeks previously. He feels unwell and his right eye is closing (**Fig. 23.1**).

The presentation of *acute* infection, as demonstrated by Peter, is very different from *chronic* infection.

List four symptoms and signs specific to each type of infection

Acute:
sick, upset child
raised temperature
red, swollen face
regional lymphodenopathy.
Chronic:
buccal sinus may be present
mobile tooth
halitosis
discoloured tooth.

Acute infections tend to present with facial cellulitis rather than a facial abscess with pus. Peter was febrile although he was not in any significant pain because the infection had perforated the cortical plate. The mainstay of treatment is removal of the cause—either pulpal extirpation or removal of the tooth.

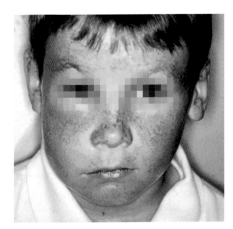

Fig. 23.1 Severe infection of canine fossa.

History

Peter traumatized his upper right lateral incisor 3 weeks ago, sustaining a deep enamel dentine fracture. The dentine was dressed with calcium hydroxide and a compomer dressing was placed over the exposed dentine and enamel. He had a review appointment with his dentist the following week.

On Saturday morning his mother noticed that his cheek was becoming swollen and the tissues around his right eye 'puffy and red'. He attended the accident and emergency department of the local hospital where he was prescribed amoxicillin 250 mg tablets to be taken three times daily for 5 days. Unfortunately, by Sunday evening Peter had become listless and his swelling had increased. He felt hot.

Examination

Extraorally there was facial asymmetry with a swelling of the right maxillary canine fossa. The overlying skin was red and hot. The right eye fissure was partially closed. Peter's temperature was 39°C. Maxillary canine fossa infections can spread via emissary veins, which have no valves, to the intracranial venous system causing either a cavernous sinus thrombosis or a brain abscess. The pathways of the IIIrd and VIth cranial nerves lie in the walls of the cavernous sinus. Thrombosis in the cavernous sinus can present with a squint due to involvement of the IIIrd and VIth cranial nerves, which are involved in control of the extraocular muscles.

What is the major problem with mandibular infections?

Spread alongside the fascial planes that surround the airway with subsequent narrowing of the airway and stridor.
Spread via the fascial planes to the mediastinum to cause a mediastinitis.

What is the basic management of any infection?

Removal of the cause—extraction or root canal therapy.
Local drainage and debridement—via root canal or incision and drainage.
Oral antibiotics if systemic involvement—amoxicillin or penicillin V are usually the drugs of first choice. Amoxicillin has the advantage that it is given with food and only needs to be taken three times per day. Metronidazole, which is active against anaerobes, can be added to either amoxicillin or penicillin if the infection is severe. Often the extraction of the abscessed tooth alone will bring about resolution without antibiotic therapy. It is important that antibiotics alone should not be considered as a first line of treatment unless there

is systemic involvement. In a child a temperature of 39°C or higher can be considered significant (normal ≅37°C). Immunosuppressed patients, or those with cardiac disease, should receive antibiotics immediately if any infection is suspected.

What are the criteria for hospital admission with orofacial infection?

Dehydration. Ask whether the child has had a decreased frequency of micturition in previous 12 hours.

Significant infection or temperature greater than 39°C.

Floor of mouth swelling.

What will the hospital management of a severe infection involve?

Extraction of involved teeth. It is impossible to drain a significant infection solely through the root canals of a tooth.

Drainage of any pus. In addition to extractions there may be a need to incise and drain pus, often leaving a drain in situ for a few days to enhance drainage. With severe mandibular swellings or where the floor of the mouth is raised, it may be necessary to have an extraoral drain through a skin incision or a 'through and through' drain, which passes completely through the area of infection. Extraoral incisions are to be avoided if at all possible due to postoperative scarring.

Swabs of pus for laboratory culture to establish accurate sensitivities of the organisms concerned to common antibiotics.

Intravenous antibiotics. Benzyl penicillin is the drug of first choice or amoxicillin. Cephalosporins are effective if there is a penicillin allergy but there is some cross-allergenicity in those patients allergic to penicillin and so cephalosporins should be used with care, especially when there was a severe reaction to penicillin. In severe infections metronidazole should be added as anaerobic organisms play a significant role.

Maintenance fluids will be given until the child is drinking normally again.

Warm saline mouthwashes.

Adequate pain control commonly with paracetamol or ibuprofen (**Table 23.1**).

If the eye is shut due to a swelling in the canine fossa it may be necessary to give chloramphenicol eye drops 0.5%, or chloramphenicol ointment 1.0% to prevent conjunctivitis.

Key point

Hospital admission in orofacial infection is necessary with:
● Dehydration.
● Temperature > 39°C.
● Floor of mouth swelling.

Treatment

Peter was treated by the following regime:

1. Extirpation of 2⌋ . The apex was not quite fully mature and good drainage of pus was achieved down the root canal.
2. Open drainage of the tooth for 2 days.
3. Amoxicillin 250 mg tds, metronidazole 200 mg bd—5 days each.
4. Hot saline mouthwashes.

After 2 days he was reviewed. The swelling was virtually absent from his right cheek and his right eye was normal. The 2⌋ was cleaned and filed and non-setting calcium hydroxide placed into the canal via a flexible tip. The access cavity was sealed with cotton wool and glass ionomer cement (GIC). The non-setting calcium hydroxide was replaced every 3 months until apical closure was achieved after 9 months. The tooth was obturated with gutta percha.

Recommended reading

Cameron A, Widmer R (eds) 2003 Paediatric oral medicine and pathology. In: Handbook of pediatric dentistry, 2nd edn. St Louis, Mosby-Wolfe, pp 140–145; 388–389.

For revision see Mind Map 23, page 169

Table 23.1 Common antibiotics and analgesics used in paediatric dentistry

Drug	Route	Dose	Frequency	Notes
Antibiotics				
Amoxycillin	PO	25–50 mg/kg/day	tds	Syrup or chewable tablets for young children
	IV	100–400 mg/kg/day	tds	
	PO, IV	50 mg/kg up to adult dose 3 g	1 hour before	Endocarditis prophylaxis. For highly susceptible patients, half dose 6 hours late
Amoxycillin plus clavulanic acid	PO	20–40 mg/kg/day	tds	For beta-lactam-resistant organisms only
Ampicillin	IV	50–100 mg/kg/day	qds	
	IV	50 mg/kg	stat	Endocarditis prophylaxis
Benzylpenicillin	IV	15–350 mg/kg/day		
		20 000–500 000 U/kg/day	qds	First IV drug of choice for odontogenic infections
Penicillin VK	PO	< 5 years 500 mg/day		
		> 5 years 1–2 g/day	qds	Give 1 hour before meals
Cephalexin	PO	25–50 mg/kg/day	qds	
Cephazolin	IV	25–50 mg/kg/day		
Erythromycin	PO	25–40 mg/kg/day	qds	Ethylsuccinate is readily absorbed
Metronidazole	IV	22.5 mg/kg/day	tds	Not in pregnancy
	PO	10–15 mg/kg/day	tds	
Gentamycin	IV	2.5 mg/kg (children) up to 80 mg maximum	stat	Endocarditis prophylaxis in highly susceptible patients in conjunction with ampicillin. Follow-up dose of ampicillin or amoxicillin required 6 hours later
Clindamycin	PO, IV	15–40 mg/kg/day	qds	Risk of pseudo-membranous colitis
	PO, IV	10 mg/kg up to adult dose 600 mg	oral 1 hour before, IV stat	Endocarditis prophylaxis. Susceptible patients. Follow-up dose half initial dose, 6 hours later (5 mg/kg up to 300 mg)
Vancomycin	IV	20 mg/kg up to adult dose 1 g	infused over 1 hour	Endocarditis prophylaxis, susceptible patients allergic to penicillin
Analgesics and sedatives				
Aspirin				Should not be used in children under 6 years of age because of the risk of Reye's syndrome
Paracetamol	PO, PR	15 mg/kg	4-hrly	Hepatotoxic if overdose
Codeine phosphate	PO	1–1.5 mg/kg single dose		
		1–3 mg/kg/day	4–6 hrly divided doses	Similar side-effects to narcotics, including nausea and constipation
Pethidine	IV, IM	1 mg/kg	3–4 hrly	Maximum 100 mg
Ibuprofen	PO	6–12 months 50 mg (5–10 mg/kg)	tds	
		1–3 yr 100 mg	tds	
		4–6 yr 150 mg	tds	
		7–9 yr 200 mg	tds	

24

The displaced primary incisor

Summary

James, who is 3, tripped over whilst playing outside. He hit his front teeth on the ground. How do you manage the immediate problem and what do you advise his parents about potential damage to the permanent teeth?

History

● Complaint

James has been brought to your surgery straight from home by his mother. She says his upper front tooth has been pushed back (**Fig. 24.1**).

● History of complaint

James tripped and fell forward hitting his teeth on the ground. One tooth is 'pushed backwards'.

● Medical history

James is a healthy boy who has had no significant childhood illnesses and who is up-to-date with all his vaccinations.

● Dental history

James has been a regular attender at his dentist since the age of 2. He has had his teeth polished and has no caries.

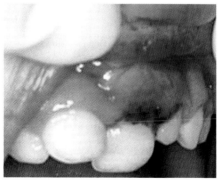

Fig. 24.1 Palatal luxation of |a .

What specific questions would you ask and why?

Was there any loss of consciousness? If there was, then this signifies intracranial trauma and the child should be referred to an accident and emergency department.

When did the accident occur? Delay in seeking help might arouse suspicions of a non-accidental injury.

Where did the accident occur? An accident outside raises the additional problem of potential wound contamination. Any child brought up in the UK should be immunized against tetanus. If a child has not been immunized seek the advice of the local GP or accident and emergency department.

What was the surface on which the accident occurred? Newly constructed playgrounds have to conform to British Standards and should be either of an energy-absorbing polymer or bark chippings. Older playgrounds and normal pathways will have non-yielding surfaces and are likely to produce greater damage and potentially greater risk of more underlying injuries.

How did the accident occur? This gives an indication of the force that produced the injury. The clinician needs to be highly suspicious of the high impact injury that looks simple. Always suspect a deeper underlying injury until proven otherwise.

Examination

● Extraoral

James is distressed but there is no obvious extraoral swelling or facial asymmetry.

● Intraoral

The appearance of the upper anterior teeth is shown in Figure 24.1. What can you see?

Palatal displacement of |1 and associated gingival trauma.

What specific signs will you look for in your examination?

The mobility of the teeth. Are they a danger to the airway?

The occlusion. Do the injured teeth prevent normal occlusion?

Mobility of a segment of teeth. This indicates a dentoalveolar fracture.

What question should dentists keep at the back of their minds when examining children?

Are the injuries consistent with the history, and if you feel they are, then is this normal behaviour?

Child physical abuse presents with orofacial signs of bruising, abrasions and lacerations, burns, bites and fractures in approximately 65% of cases.

Dentists should have a copy of their local area Child Protection Committee guidelines. This will tell them who they should contact for advice.

What features in the history and examination would lead to suspicions of child physical abuse?

There are ten items to consider. Five are questions to ask yourself and five are observations about the behaviour of the child and the parent(s):

Could the injury have been caused accidentally and if so how?

Does the explanation for the injury fit the age and the clinical findings?

If the explanation of the cause is consistent with the injury, is this itself within the normally acceptable limits of behaviour?

If there has been delay in seeking advice are there good reasons for this?

Does the story of the accident vary?

The nature of the relationship between parent and child.

The child's reactions to other people.

The child's reactions to any medical or dental examinations.

The general demeanour of the child.

Any comments made by the child and/or parent that give concern about the child's upbringing or lifestyle.

Investigations
What investigations would you perform for James? Explain why for each

Radiographs are required to visualize the traumatized area and assess whether there are any root fractures to either the traumatized or adjacent teeth. In addition, is a dentoalveolar fracture evident? Are permanent successor teeth present? In an intrusive injury a child may have been referred as an 'avulsed' incisor. It is imperative always to check in these circumstances that the tooth is not intruded. Re-eruption of an intruded tooth may occur and close review is necessary. If re-eruption has not occurred within 4–6 months an intruded primary incisor should be removed to minimize eruptive problems in the permanent dentition. An adult periapical film used as an anterior occlusal is the easiest way to obtain a periapical view of the upper anterior region in a young child. James's radiograph did not reveal any root fractures or dentoalveolar fractures.

Vitality testing of primary teeth is not indicated.

Diagnosis
What is your diagnosis?

James has a palatal luxation injury to his upper left primary central incisor.

Treatment
What are the three key components of the history and examination in primary tooth trauma that will dictate if active treatment is required?

Pain. Either spontaneous or on eating suggests pathosis.

Mobility. Is the tooth a danger to the airway?

Occlusal interference. A luxation injury that has prevented normal intercuspal occlusion will prevent normal eating.

What treatments are usually required for displaced primary incisors?

Concussion and subluxation: observation.

Lateral luxation: if no occlusal interference, the tooth is allowed to reposition spontaneously; if occlusal interference – extract.

Intrusion: if the apex is displaced toward the labial bone plate, then leave for spontaneous repositioning. If no movement within 4–6 months, extract. If the apex is displaced into the developing toothgerm, extract.

Extrusion: extract or reposition if only a minor extrusion.

Avulsion: replantation is not indicated.

Key point

Traumatized primary teeth may need to be extracted if:
● Pain interrupts eating or sleeping.
● Excessive mobility causes a danger to the airway.
● There is occlusal interference.

What radiographs would you take for these displacement injuries?

Concussion and subluxation: periapical.

Lateral luxation: occlusal view shows increased periodontal space apically.

Intrusion: periapical and extraoral lateral.

Extrusion: periapical.

Avulsion: periapical to ensure that missing tooth is not intruded.

What are you going to tell James's mother about the risk to the permanent teeth?

The reported incidences of damage to the developing permanent teeth as a result of trauma to primary incisors range from 17% to 64%. An easily remembered figure to tell all parents at the time of the initial presentation would be 50%. It is better to be pessimistic and then be pleasantly surprised on eruption of the permanent teeth rather than the opposite.

What are the possible effects on the permanent successor teeth?

White or yellow-brown discolouration of enamel (hypomineralization).
Enamel hypoplasia.
Crown dilaceration.
Crown–root dilaceration.
Root dilaceration.
Odontome formation.
Partial/complete arrest of root formation.
Sequestration of permanent toothgerm.
Disturbance in eruption.

Can you tell all of these sequelae on a periapical radiograph?

No. Only structural abnormalities and abnormal root growth will be visible. White and brown areas of hypomineralization will only be evident on eruption of the permanent teeth.

If you retain a luxated primary tooth how often would you review it?

One week after the injury, 1 month, then 3-monthly.

How would you review it?

Historically: symptoms.
Clinically: colour, sinus, tenderness.
Radiographically: 6-monthly if possible.

Key point

After primary tooth trauma:
- Damage to permanent teeth may occur in 50% of cases.
- Intrusive trauma causes most permanent tooth damage.

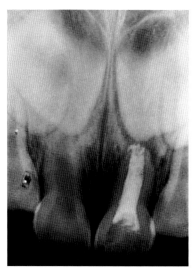

Fig. 24.2 Endodontically treated primary incisor.

Does a discoloured primary incisor always need treatment?

When there is progressive worsening of discolouration then the tooth will be non-vital. When there is a grey discolouration that does not get worse then vitality may be maintained. In the absence of periapical pathosis a discoloured primary incisor can be reviewed. In the presence of pathosis then either extraction or root canal therapy with zinc oxide paste is indicated (**Fig. 24.2**).

Recommended reading

Curzon MEJ (ed) 1999 Handbook of dental trauma. Wright, Oxford.
Roberts G, Longhurst P 1996 Oral and dental trauma in children and adolescents. Oxford University Press, Oxford.
Welbury RR (ed) Traumatic injuries to the teeth. In: Paediatric dentistry, 2nd edn. Oxford University Press, Oxford.

For revision see Mind Map 24, page 170

25

The fractured immature permanent incisor crown

Summary

Shay is 8. Whilst saving a penalty for his school team he collided with the goal post and sustained enamel dentine pulp and enamel dentine fractures to his upper central incisors. How would you manage the injuries, and outline a follow-up treatment plan?

History
● Complaint

The upper right and left central permanent incisors are fractured (**Fig. 25.1**).

● History of complaint

The injury was sustained during a game of soccer. There were no other injuries.

● Medical history

Shay is a healthy boy with no history of illness. He has had all his vaccinations including a preschool booster for tetanus.

● Dental history

Shay is a regular attender at his dentist and has had local anaesthetic for a restoration.

What specific questions would you ask and why?

Was there any loss of consciousness?
Was the fractured piece of tooth located?

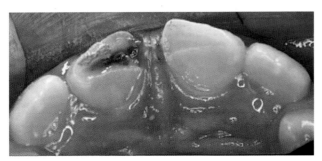

Fig. 25.1 Trauma to the central incisors.

A history of loss of consciousness together with a missing tooth fragment is an indication for a chest radiograph to check that there has not been inhalation of the tooth fragment.

When did the injury occur?
The time from the injury to presentation may affect the treatment options.

Did Shay cope well with his previous experience of local anaesthetic?
The answer to this will dictate what treatment strategies will be possible.

Examination
● Extraoral
Why is the presence of lip swelling together with a mucosal laceration important?

This could indicate that the missing tooth fragment is retained in the lip.

How would you demonstrate there was a fragment of tooth in the lip?

By soft tissue radiography using two views at right angles to each other. A simple anteroposterior view using a periapical film placed behind the lip and in front of the teeth, followed by a lateral soft tissue view using a lateral occlusal film (**Fig. 25.2**). Clinically, a fragment of tooth is often best located by 'feel' with a probe.

Key point

Missing tooth fragments could:
● Be within the soft tissues if there is a laceration.
● Have been inhaled if there was loss of consciousness.

● Intraoral
What injuries are visible in Figure 25.1*?*

There is an enamel dentine fracture of $\underline{1}$ and an enamel dentine pulp fracture of $1\underline{|}$ of greater than 1 mm in diameter.

Are the roots of the 1| and |1 likely to have open or closed apices?

Open. Apices are not usually closed on upper permanent central incisors before the age of 11 years.

How would you confirm apical status?
Periapical radiograph.

What other injuries must you exclude on the periapical radiograph?

Root fractures.

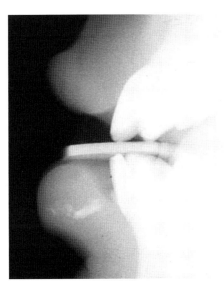

Fig. 25.2 Fragments of tooth in lower lip (different case).

What other features of the anterior teeth are important at examination?

Mobility. In a buccopalatal direction. Excessive mobility suggests either a periodontal ligament injury or a root fracture.

Colour. This will indicate whether any direct pulpal damage causing haemorrhage into the dentinal tubules has occurred.

Percussion. Tenderness suggests periapical damage and oedema. A dull note may suggest a clinically undiagnosed vertical crown fracture or root fracture.

Vitality. Following trauma there may be a period of apparent loss of vitality on testing with hot and cold stimuli or the electric pulp tester even in teeth without obvious crown fractures. Nevertheless, the readings serve as a baseline against which subsequent tests can be compared.

What teeth should be examined after trauma affecting only upper centrals?

All upper and lower incisors should be included in an examination after any trauma to the anterior region.

Investigations

Radiographs (previously mentioned) for:
Foreign body in soft tissues if applicable.
Apical status of teeth.
Presence or absence of root fractures.
Vitality testing of all upper and lower incisors.

Treatment

What is the prime consideration for both the upper central incisors?

To maintain vital pulp within the root, which will allow physiological dentine deposition resulting in full root growth and a root with a normal dentinal wall thickness which will not be prone to fracture.

What is the appropriate immediate treatment for the ⌊1 that has an enamel dentine fracture?

Reattachment of the fragment, or

A bonded restoration/'bandage', which will produce a hermetic seal. Glass ionomer cement is not an adequate material for a 'bandage' and will fracture or be lost resulting in thermal damage to the pulp from hot and cold stimuli. A layer of setting calcium hydroxide cement should be placed over dentine where a pulpal shadow is visible prior to placement of an adhesive bandage.

What are the treatment options for the 1⌋ that has a pulpal exposure?

Direct pulp capping; complete pulpotomy; partial pulpotomy. Direct pulp capping, the placement of wound dressings on an exposed pulp, is considered very unpredictable by many authors. Partial pulpotomy (subtotal or Cvek) is the removal of only the outer layer of damaged and hyperaemic tissue in the exposed pulps and will also allow continued full root growth. Partial pulpotomy is a highly successful technique. Complete pulpotomy (cervical pulpotomy) is the removal of coronal pulp tissue and the placement of a wound dressing on the canal orifice. Complete pulpotomy will arrest dentine formation in the pulp chamber but allow full root growth. Complete endodontic treatment will then only be necessary in the future if the root canal is required for retention of a coronal restoration.

What are the indications for permanent tooth partial pulpotomy?

No history of spontaneous pain.
Acute minor pain that subsides with analgesics.
No discomfort to percussion, no sulcus swelling, no mobility.
Radiographic examination shows normal periodontal ligament.
Pulp is exposed during caries removal or subsequent to recent trauma.
Tissue appears vital.
Bleeding from the pulp excision site stops with isotonic saline irrigation within 2 minutes.

How would you carry out a partial pulpotomy?

Local analgesia.
Rubber dam.
Smooth sharp fracture edges or remaining carious dentine.
Flush exposed pulp with isotonic saline solution.

Superficial layer of exposed pulp and surrounding dentine are excised to about 2 mm using a high-speed diamond bur with light touch under waterspray cooling.

Surface of remaining pulp is irrigated gently with isotonic saline until bleeding has ceased.

Apply a pulpal medicament with biologically available calcium hydroxide and seal coronal cavity with a bonded restoration.

Care should be taken to avoid a significant blood clot developing between the wound surface and the dressing medicament. Dry, sterile cotton pellets are used carefully to adapt the calcium hydroxide medicament to the prepared cavity. The bonded restoration will ensure that there will be no bacterial leakage into the tooth following restoration.

The time from injury to presentation for treatment has been reported to be important with regard to the success of partial pulpotomy, with treatment within 24 hours giving the best results. However, proper treatment of pulp tissue and careful case selection are likely to be the key issues for a good outcome. Pulp tissue compromised by infection and inflammation must be removed to facilitate physiological haemostasis during saline irrigation. The larger and the deeper an access cavity needs to be to reach healthy tissue the more likelihood there is of widespread infection and thus suggests a likely clinical contraindication to vital pulp therapy.

How should the crown of 1| be restored?

If the crown fragment has been retrieved then this can be stored in normal saline whilst the partial (subtotal) pulpotomy is completed. The fragment can then be reattached.

If the crown fragment is not available or the fracture extends significantly subgingivally then a bonded composite restoration should be provided.

Figures 25.3 and **25.4** show the crown fragments before and after reattachment in Shay's case. 1| had a partial pulpotomy as described.

How should the upper centrals be reviewed and how often?

Definitive crown morphology should be restored as soon as possible after emergency treatment to re-establish normal sagittal relations with the lower incisors.

One-, 3-, and then 6-monthly clinical and radiographic examination to check for continued vitality and normal root growth. If there is

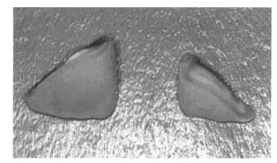

Fig. 25.3 Fragments found at scene of incident.

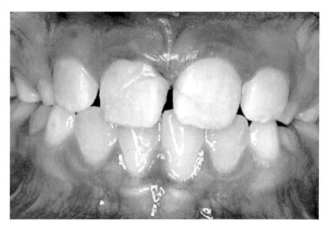

Fig. 25.4 Fragments reattached.

Key point

Partial or complete pulpotomy:
- Has a high success rate.
- Is more successful if completed within 24 hours of an injury.
- Allows full root growth with a vital radicular pulp.

evidence of non-vitality then the immature tooth must be extirpated and non-setting calcium hydroxide used to stimulate root end closure prior to obturation with gutta percha.

Recommended reading

Curzon MEJ (ed) 1999 Handbook of dental trauma. Wright, Oxford.

Roberts G, Longhurst P 1996 Oral and dental trauma in children and adolescents. Oxford University Press, Oxford.

Whitworth J, Nunn J 2001 Endodontic treatment of teeth. In: Welbury RR (ed) Paediatric dentistry, 2nd edn. Oxford University Press, Oxford.

For revision see Mind Map 25, page 171

26

The fractured permanent incisor root

Summary

Andrea is 12. She was trampolining at school when she fell and sustained middle third root fractures of 1| and |1. How do you manage this type of injury, and what do you advise her about the long-term prognosis for those teeth?

History

● Complaint

Andrea is brought to your surgery by a schoolteacher. She is complaining that her upper permanent central incisors are loose and feel 'funny' when she bites together.

● History of complaint

Andrea fell forward whilst on the trampoline at school and hit her teeth on the edge of the trampoline. Her mother arrives at the surgery soon after Andrea and her teacher. It appears Andrea was not being supervised on the trampoline and the foam protection was not in the correct position on the metal frame of the trampoline. Her mother is not very happy with the explanation by the teacher.

What does this alert you to?

The possibility of legal action against the school. It is especially important to make drawings of any external injuries on the face and keep accurate records of intra-oral injuries and subsequent treatment. A photographic record will be an advantage.

● Medical history

Andrea is under regular care with her dentist and has had local anaesthetic without problem.

What specific questions would you ask and why?

Was there any loss of consciousness? If there was, then Andrea should be referred to an accident and emergency department.

Is there any pain or discomfort whilst opening and closing the jaw? Absence of symptoms should rule out any condylar injury/fracture. When the force that produces an injury is significant then it should raise suspicion of a deeper underlying bony injury. Bony injury would be more likely in Andrea's case compared to the scenario of root fractures on teeth that had been produced by less force.

Examination

● Extraoral

There is some swelling of the upper lip and some bruising and swelling under the right eye.

What questions and examination would you complete regarding the swelling and bruising under the right eye?

Is there any double vision? Palpate the infraorbital margin for 'stepping' and then check for altered sensation over the distribution of the infraorbital nerve. Check that there is a full range of eye movements—especially upward gaze. Fracture of the infraorbital margin and infraorbital floor could lead to entrapment of the inferior oblique extraocular muscle preventing upward and outward movement of the globe of the eye.

Is there any altered sensation on the cheek? Oedema surrounding the infraorbital nerve or entrapment of the nerve in a fracture can result in paraesthesia.

If there is any doubt about a fracture then posteroan-terior and occipitomental views will detect displacement of the infraorbital margin, and tomograms will detect orbital floor 'blowout' fractures.

● Intraoral

There is downward and palatal displacement of the crowns of 1| and |1, which are mobile. Centric occlusion is not possible because of the slightly palatal position of 1| and |1.

What tests would you do prior to repositioning of the teeth?

Radiographs. Intraoral periapicals (**Fig. 27.1**) or an anterior occlusal view are needed to diagnose root fractures compared to luxation injuries. The upper lateral incisors 2|, |2 should also be checked for injury. Consideration should also be given to radiography of the lower incisors, which must also have received either direct or indirect trauma. Where there is no significant displacement of the coronal portion of a tooth with a root fracture, then an anterior occlusal radiograph will often detect root fractures that may not be so evident on periapical views. These radiographs will serve as baseline views prior to repositioning.

Vitality tests on all upper and lower incisors.

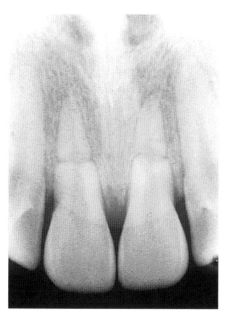

Fig. 26.1 Middle third root fractures.

Treatment

What design of splint would you use for 1|, |1? You have confirmed on radiography that they have middle third root fractures (Fig. 26.1)

The splint should be flexible/functional and designed to have one sound abutment tooth on either side of the root fractured teeth.

How long should the splint be in place?

For 2–3 weeks until the majority of periodontal ligament fibres have healed. This time can be extended if there are clinical indications for this. The old regime of rigid splinting for 2–3 months for root fractures has been shown to have no benefit. Rigid splinting was meant to give the fracture its best chance of a hard tissue union. Research has shown that hard tissue union is most likely to occur if there was little displacement at the time of the original injury rather than being a function of the type of splint employed. In other words the larger the displacement at the fracture line at the time of the injury, the smaller the chance of a hard tissue union between the fracture ends after reduction and splinting.

Do any forms of dentoalveolar injury need to be rigidly splinted?

Only dentoalveolar fractures for a duration of 3–4 weeks. A rigid splint would involve two sound abutment teeth on either side of the injury. All other displacement injuries, root fractures and avulsions require flexible/functional splints. Avulsions usually only require splinting for 7–10 days whilst the others require 2–3 weeks.

> **Key point**
>
> Splinting in dentoalveolar trauma:
> - Flexible 7–10 days for avulsions.
> - Flexible 2–3 weeks for luxations, root fractures.
> - Rigid 3–4 weeks for dentoalveolar fractures.

Describe your step by step procedure for reduction and splinting Andrea's 1| and |1.

Give topical and local anaesthetic labially and palatally.

While the local anaesthetic is taking effect bend a section of 0.6-mm stainless steel wire to the shape of the upper labial segment to include the four incisor teeth.

Gently reposition 1|, |1 and hold these in approximate position with some red wax palatally, which extends over the incisal edges 1|, |1.

Etch labial surface 2|, |2, wash, dry, place bonding resin and a spot of composite in the centre of the labial surface.

Place 0.6-mm wire into position on 2|, |2. Use a bonding brush to mould the composite already on the teeth over the wire. Add extra composite if required. Cure composite.

Remove wax and with non-working hand bring 1|, |1 into an accurate position against the wire splint. Hold them in this position whilst etching, washing, bonding and adding composite with working hand. Cure composite.

Smooth any rough areas with soflex discs.

On removal of the splint how often would you review Andrea?

After 1 month, then 3 months and finally 6-monthly.

What tests would you complete at each of these reviews?

For all traumatized teeth a regime should be followed. If this is done in every case then omissions are less likely to be made.

Clinical:
colour (palatal surface best)
buccal sulcus sensitivity to digital pressure
sinus presence
tenderness to percussion
mobility
sensibility testing.
Radiography: long cone periapicals.

Is sensibility testing accurate?

No form of sensibility testing on its own is accurate. Electric pulp testing (EPT) is probably the most accurate but its real value lies in successive numerical readings with the same type of EPT. Numerical values can then be compared. In the future the widespread use of Doppler in detecting blood flow in a traumatized tooth will inform all decisions regarding pulpal necrosis and the necessity for extirpation.

Key point
What types of healing occur in root fractures?
● Hard tissue.
● Connective tissue.
● Osseous.

What is the likely radiographic appearance at the fracture line if the coronal tooth portion becomes non-vital?

There will be increasing widening and translucency between the fractured ends of root.

If the coronal portion of an apical or middle third root fractured tooth became non-vital, how would you root treat the tooth?

Extirpation to the fracture line.
Establish working length to fracture line.
Place non-setting calcium hydroxide 1 mm short of fracture line with aim of inducing barrier formation.
Change non-setting calcium hydroxide 3-monthly until barrier forms.
Obturate with gutta percha to barrier.
Annual radiographic review.

What happens to the apical fragment?

In nearly all cases this will undergo intracanal sclerosis and will not need treatment. If there is infection of the apical fragment then it may require surgical removal. Root canal therapy across a root fracture is fraught with difficulty because of problems keeping the distal canal dry.

Is the prognosis good in coronal or gingival third root fractures?

No. Decisions need to be made early regarding options. Long-term stability and long-term retention of the whole tooth in these injuries is rare.

What are the treatment options in coronal or gingival third root fractures?

Retain crown temporarily with an endodontic post across the fracture line.
Remove coronal fragment. Root treat apical fragment and orthodontically extrude prior to post, core and crown placement.
Remove coronal fragment. Root treat apical fragment

and cover with a mucoperiosteal flap. The width and height of the alveolus are thus retained for future implant placement. Prosthetic replacement required. Remove all portions of tooth. Prosthetic replacement required. Future implant placement.

Can root fractured teeth maintain vitality?

Yes. The majority do so. **Figures 26.2** and **26.3** show Andrea's teeth 3 years after the original injury. The teeth maintained vitality and underwent progressive intra-canal sclerosis. In addition the distal fragments are resorbing. Importantly, there has been no infection.

Can root fractured teeth be moved orthodontically?

Yes, but with caution. If there is not a hard tissue union between the fracture ends then the apical portion will remain static and only the coronal portion will move. Regular radiographic review is necessary during any orthodontic treatment.

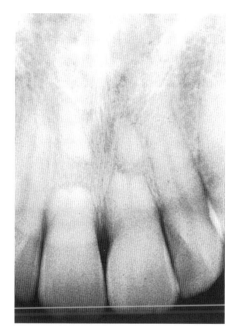

Fig. 26.2 Radiographic appearance after 3 years.

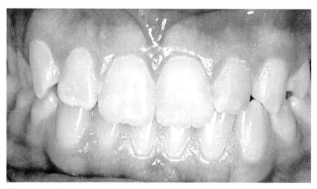

Fig. 26.3 Clinical appearance after 3 years.

Recommended reading

Curzon MEJ (ed) 1999 Handbook of dental trauma. Wright, Oxford.

Roberts G, Longhurst P 1996 Oral and dental trauma in children and adolescents. Oxford University Press, Oxford.

Welbury RR (ed) Traumatic injuries to the teeth. In: Paediatric dentistry, 2nd edn. Oxford University Press, Oxford:.

For revision see Mind Map 26, page 172

27

The avulsed incisor

Summary

Kathryn is 9. She was playing with her friends at Brownie camp with a skipping rope, when the rope caught behind one of her upper central incisors and avulsed it. Her teacher has got the tooth. How would you manage this problem?

Kathryn's teacher phones your surgery for advice. She has the tooth in a handkerchief. The accident was 10 minutes ago. What is your advice?

Check Kathryn has no other injuries, i.e. head injuries that require referral to an accident and emergency department.

Check for any known medical history.

Hold tooth by crown, wash gently under cold water to remove any debris for 10 seconds.

Replant in socket ideally.

Hold tooth in socket by biting on a handkerchief. Come to surgery.

If replantation not possible, place tooth in either milk or normal saline (First Aid box) and bring to surgery with Kathryn.

The tooth is brought to the surgery in milk. How would you proceed?

Check medical history. Heart defects, immunosuppression and a history of rheumatic fever are reasons to not consider replantation.

Place tooth in normal saline. Remove any foreign bodies. Check state of root development.

Labial and palatal local anaesthetic.

Irrigate socket with normal saline.

Recontour labial plate with flat plastic instrument or Couplands elevator, if required.

Gently but firmly reposition avulsed tooth.

Bend a 0.6-mm stainless steel wire to include one tooth either side of avulsed tooth.

Follow guidelines in Chapter 26 for placement of the splint.

Prescribe chlorhexidine mouthwash and antibiotics. Amoxycillin 125 mg tds for 5 days is an appropriate antibiotic. If allergic to amoxycillin

then use erythromycin 125 mg qds for 5 days. Chlorhexidine 0.2% should be used twice daily to help normal oral hygiene.

Arrange a review appointment for 7–10 days.

What factors are important when deciding whether root canal treatment is necessary in Kathryn's case?

Apical development.

The time that the tooth was out of the mouth (extra alveolar time).

A tooth that has a mature apex will rarely undergo revascularization. The only tooth that has a chance of revascularization is the immature tooth with an open apex that is replanted within 30–45 minutes. All other teeth apart from the immature apex replanted within 30–45 minutes should be extirpated prior to splint removal at 7–10 days.

What intracanal medicament should be placed in the extirpated tooth?

There has been some in-vitro work that has shown that if non-setting calcium hydroxide is inadvertently spun through the apex of a tooth with a damaged periodontal ligament (PL), then instead of normal repair of PL fibres there may be replacement resorption. With this in mind some authorities advocate that Ledermix/Polyantibiotic paste should be the first dressing placed in root canals of teeth with PL injuries if extirpation occurs within 14 days of the injury. However, other authorities claim that the above research has never been shown to be a real risk in vivo and, therefore, place non-setting calcium hydroxide as the initial dressing to a calculated working length.

What factors are important in predicting resorption?

Extra alveolar dry time (EADT).

Total extra alveolar time (EAT).

Recent research has shown that teeth with a dry time of greater than 15 minutes have a significantly increased risk of resorption. The two preferred storage media, milk and normal saline, are iso-osmolar and that is why they are recommended storage media. However, the PL cannot retain vitality for long periods even in these media.

What types of resorption are there?

Surface: normally seen as blunting of tooth apices after application of excessive orthodontic forces or on the roots of upper lateral incisors as a result of canine tooth impaction. The teeth are usually vital in surface resorption.

External inflammatory: initiated in the PL after traumatic injury. The surfaces of the roots have punched-out craters where multipotent PL cells have become osteoclastic and started resorbing cementum and dentine. The walls of the root canal are intact. Exacerbated by a non-vital pulp.

Internal inflammatory: originating in the root canal. Usually due to inadequate mechanical and chemical debridement of a non-vital tooth.

Replacement: external replacement resorption is characterized by absence of PL and bone is fused to cementum and dentine. The tooth becomes part of bone and is constantly remodelled, resulting in progressive resorption of the root. In traumatology, external replacement resorption will inevitably follow external inflammatory resorption where there has been permanent damage to the PL. Internal replacement resorption or progressive pulp canal obliteration or sclerosis is the response of a vital pulp to trauma.

Key point

Critical historical information in avulsion:
- EADT.
- EAT.
- Storage medium.

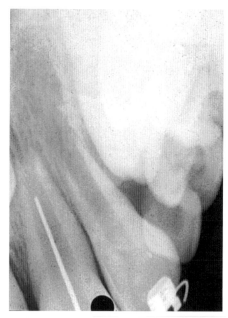

Fig. 27.1 Replanted incisor at pulp extirpation.

What is the treatment if inflammatory resorption occurs after trauma?

The only medicament we have that has the potential to stop the inflammatory resorption is non-setting calcium hydroxide. It is alkaline (pH 11–12), antibacterial and anti-inflammatory. It should be replaced within the root canal every 3–6 months, either until resorption has halted and a gutta percha root filling can be placed, or the tooth is lost as a result of progressive resorption.

Kathryn's |1 had an EADT of 10 minutes. Her tooth was then placed in milk and brought to the surgery prior to reimplantation. The total EAT was 1 hour 50 minutes. The tooth was extirpated prior to splint removal at 10 days and non-setting calcium hydroxide placed in the root canal (**Fig. 27.1**). A normal PL reformed and there was continued apexification and apical development as a result of 3-monthly changes in non-setting calcium hydroxide (**Fig. 27.2**). The tooth was subsequently obturated with gutta percha and should be retained as a functioning unit for life.

If resorption in |1 was progressive how would you plan for its ultimate loss?

Try to maintain |1 for as long as possible as its presence helps to maintain both the height and the width of the alveolus. This will be important in future prosthetic considerations.

Replace |1 with an immediate replacement denture when it is eventually lost. Maintain the denture until upper canines have erupted.

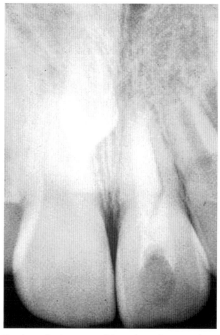

Fig. 27.2 Root end closure achieved and normal periodontal ligament.

Resin-retained bridge to replace |1 until 18 years of age.

Consideration for single osseo-integrated implant at age 18–20.

Key point

Types of resorption:
- Surface.
- Inflammatory—external and internal.
- Replacement—external and internal.

How does the EADT influence your treatment of the avulsed incisor?

Recent guidelines would suggest that 60 minutes is a critical time. If a tooth has been dry for less than 60 minutes then the PL has potential to survive and conventional treatments should be followed including splinting for 7–10 days and elective extirpation prior to splint removal for all teeth except the tooth with an immature apex that has been out of the mouth for less than 30–45 minutes.

If a tooth has been kept dry for greater than 60 minutes then the following treatment should be instituted. If the apex is very immature then the tooth should not be reimplanted. In this circumstance the risks of ankylosis and resorption are high and the tooth will be lost quickly from the mouth. This is due to the high turnover rate of bone at this age. If the apex is mature then the PL should be scraped off the root with a sharp excavator and the tooth either immersed in 2.4% sodium fluoride solution, acidulated to pH 5.5 for 5 minutes prior to reimplantation. The sodium fluoride solution will increase the resistance of the root to future resorption. In these cases where the PL is removed prior to reimplantation, it is optional whether extirpation and obturation is done extraorally or once the tooth has been repositioned. Splinting after PL removal should be for 2–3 months.

Recommended reading

Curzon MEJ (ed) Handbook of dental trauma. Wright, Oxford.
Gregg TA, Boyd DH 1998 UK National Clinical Guideline. Treatment of avulsed permanent teeth in children. Int J Paediatr Dent 8:75–81.
Roberts G, Longhurst P 1996 Oral and dental trauma in children and adolescents. Oxford University Press, Oxford.

For revision see Mind Map 27, page 173

28

Poor quality first permanent molars

Summary

Lisa is 9. Her mother has brought her to your surgery because her new permanent teeth at the back of her mouth are brown and there are white and brown patches on her new incisors. What has caused these discolourations? How may they be treated?

History

Lisa has complained that for the past few months the teeth have been painful on eating hot and cold foods. The pain is of 1–2 minutes' duration. Toothbrushing also has caused sensitivity at the back of the mouth. There has been no pain on biting and eating foods. Very recently Lisa felt that one of the back teeth especially has started to crumble. Her mother has also noticed this when she has helped with brushing.

Lisa has not required any analgesics for the discomfort caused by her teeth.

● Medical history

Lisa is a healthy child who has never been in hospital.

● Dental history

Lisa and her family are regular dental attenders. The family all have a low caries risk. Lisa has no restorations in her primary dentition. She used a children's toothpaste (500 ppm) until recently and is now on the same adult paste as her parents (1450 ppm).

Examination

Intraoral examination revealed that all four first permanent molars (FPMs) were hypomineralized with areas of brown, rough enamel. In addition there were areas of hypoplasia where the enamel had chipped away exposing underlying dentine. The maxillary molars were the worst affected by hypoplasia. $\overline{6|}$ had a large amalgam restoration. In addition some white and brown hypomineralized areas were visible on the labial surfaces of the newly erupted upper and lower permanent central incisors (**Figs 28.1** and **28.2**).

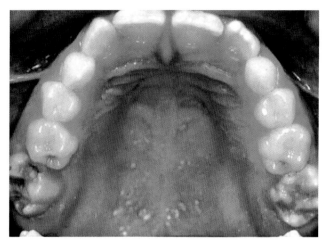

Fig. 28.1 Hypomineralized and hypoplastic upper first permanent molars.

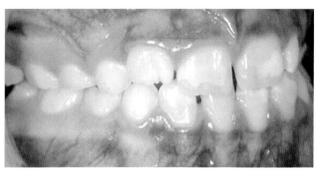

Fig. 28.2 Hypomineralized upper and lower permanent incisors.

'Hypomineralized' is the name given to enamel when it has a reduced mineral content. 'Hypoplasia' is the name applied when there is a reduced thickness of enamel.

Upper and lower arches were uncrowded. Space assessed from the distal of 2's to mesial of 6's in each quadrant was 21.5 mm in the lower arch and 22 mm in each upper arch quadrant. On average, 21 mm and 22 mm are required for these distances in the lower and upper arches, respectively.

The incisor relationship was just Class I on $\underline{1|1}$; the molar relationship was Class I bilaterally.

Do you think that the enamel hypomineralization and hypoplasia noted on the first permanent molars and the permanent incisors follows a chronological pattern? If so at what time was the affected enamel formed?

Yes, it is possible that there is a chronological pattern. The cusp tips of the first permanent molars begin mineralizing from the eighth month of pregnancy. The cusp tips of the incisors and cuspids (canines) from about 3 months of age (the upper lateral incisor is slightly later at 10–12 months). Mineralization dates for the permanent dentition are given in Table 28.1.

Table 28.1 Mineralization times for the permanent dentition

Tooth	Mineralization begins (months)
Upper	
Central incisor	3–4
Lateral incisor	10–12
Canine	4–5
First premolar	18–21
Second premolar	24–27
First molar	at birth
Second molar	30–36
Third molar	84–108
Lower	
Central incisor	3–4
Lateral incisor	3–4
Canine	4–5
First premolar	21–24
Second premolar	27–30
First molar	at birth
Second molar	30–36
Third molar	96–120

Key point

● Mineralization of FPM commences around birth.

What specific questions would you like to ask Lisa's mother?

Prenatal. Mother's health during pregnancy. Were there any concerns such as high blood pressure and proteinuria—pre-eclampsia?

Perinatal. Difficult birth. Was the delivery prolonged? Was there a need for assisted delivery by forceps, ventouse or caesarean? All of these could indicate fetal distress.

Postnatal. Did the child spend any time in the special care baby unit (SCBU)?

Illnesses in the first 2 years of life, e.g. meningitis, measles, respiratory infections.

These disturbances may manifest as enamel defects distributed in the enamel that was forming around birth and in the first 2 years of life.

Further questioning revealed that Lisa was born after a normal pregnancy and delivery but had a significant number of respiratory infections during the first year of life. This confirms your diagnosis of chronological hypoplasia. The correct name for this condition is molar incisor hypomineralization (MIH).

What other differential diagnoses might you consider?

Caries. Newly erupted teeth are particularly prone to dental caries until their enamel maturation is complete. However, it seems very unlikely, even in the presence of particularly deep fissures, that Lisa, who has no caries in her primary teeth, should develop such caries in her permanent teeth. In addition the overall colour of the permanent molars is not consistent with caries in a tooth of normal morphology. The exposed dentine is slightly softened and does have caries but the overall pattern of destruction of the tooth suggests that caries is secondary to some other predisposing factor such as hypomineralization/hypoplasia. Another factor to consider that is against a diagnosis of caries is the white hypomineralized areas on the incisors. They are neither the shape nor the distribution of white spot or precarious lesions that one would expect with poor oral hygiene.

Amelogenesis imperfecta. Although the presenting features could be a hypomature form of amelogenesis imperfecta, there are several factors that suggest this is not the case: there is no family history; the primary dentition is not affected; the pattern of the defects is chronological. All of these combined make an inherited abnormality unlikely.

Fluorosis. The defects on the molar teeth could only occur if there was a history of very high endemic fluoride levels, probably in excess of 6 ppm. Such levels do not occur in the UK. Mild fluorosis is seen where children have swallowed toothpaste or have been given supplementation in addition to swallowing toothpaste. However, in such cases there are usually fine opaque white lines following the perikymata and small irregular enamel opacities or flecks that merge into the background enamel colour. Fluorosis does not produce well-demarcated opacities like those seen on the incisors.

Key point

In MIH your questioning should include:
● Prenatal period.
● Natal period.
● Postnatal period.
● Systemic illnesses in first 2 years of life.

Is pain from such molar teeth common?

Yes. There is evidence that these teeth have 5–10 times greater treatment need than normal teeth and are more difficult to anaesthetize. A palatal as well as a buccal infiltration is often required. There is also evidence that children with hypomineralized first permanent molars (HFPMs) have more behaviour management problems than other children, necessitating adjuncts to treatment such as sedation. In recent years, the prevalence of HFPMs in Europe has been shown to be between 10% and 20% (**Table 28.2**).

The histology of extracted HFPMs shows that the yellow/brown areas are more porous and occupy the whole enamel layer. The white/cream areas occupy the inner parts of enamel. The affected areas have a higher carbon, and lower calcium and phosphate content.

Table 28.2 Prevalence of HFPMs in European studies

Country	Prevalence (%)	Age of children (years)	Year of publication
Finland	19.3	7–13	2001
The Netherlands	10	11	2000
Sweden	15.4	8–16	1987
Sweden	18.5	7–8	2001
UK	14.5	7	2002

Investigations

What investigations are indicated and why?

Intraoral radiographs are indicated in order to assess the proximity of the coronal defects to the dental pulp. A *panoramic tomogram* is necessary to ascertain the presence and stage of development of the remaining permanent dentition in view of the poor long-term prognosis of the first permanent molars.

A panoramic tomogram revealed all permanent teeth, including third molars, to be present. The furcation of 7's was calcifying. Secondary caries was evident in all first permanent molars but was most pronounced in $\frac{6|6}{|6}$.

Treatment

What are the main clinical problems in this case?

Loss of tooth substance:
    breakdown of enamel
    tooth wear
    secondary caries.
Sensitivity.
Appearance.

Key point

Children with MIH:
● Have a higher treatment need.
● Have significantly higher behaviour management problems.

What are the treatment options for the HFPMs in this case?

Composite/glass ionomer cement (GIC) restorations.
Stainless steel crowns.
Adhesively retained copings.
Extraction.

● Composite/GIC restorations

These can be definitive restorations when the area of hypomineralization does not involve a cusp, or temporizing restorations. It is important when restoring these teeth that all the hypomineralized area is removed.

● Stainless steel crowns

These are the most durable restoration and can maintain a tooth until a permanent crown can be placed in teenage years, or until a planned extraction.

● Adhesively retained copings

These may be suitable for teeth that are not significantly affected by hypomineralization. When the defect has been removed and replaced by GIC then a coping can be placed on top of the restoration and covering the remainder of the occlusal and cuspal surface.

● Extraction

This is the preferred treatment option because HFPMs:
1. Are of poor long-term prognosis. Although full coverage coronal restorations could be undertaken to retain them, this is an ambitious plan in a 9-year-old child. The restorations undoubtedly would require replacement at some future date due to possible microleakage at the margins and caries. This would incur additional inconvenience and expense to the patient.
2. It is the optimal developmental stage to remove $\overline{6}$'s as the furcation of $\overline{7}$'s is calcifying and bodily movement of $\overline{7}$ forward will be encouraged. Timing of $\overline{6}$ removal is more critical than that of $\underline{6}$ as the mesial drift tendency is greater in the upper arch.

Third molar teeth are also developing and should erupt eventually if 7's migrate forward to occupy the position of the 6's (Fig. 28.3).
3. As the molar relationship is Class I bilaterally, removal of $\overline{6}$'s necessitates the removal of $\underline{6}$'s to encourage maintenance of the buccal segment relationship. This is known as balancing (removal of a tooth from the opposite side of the arch) and compensating (removal of the equivalent opposing tooth) extractions.

For revision see Mind Map 28, page 174

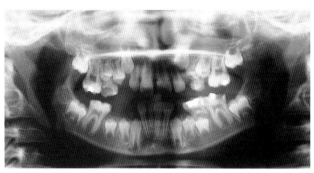

Fig. 28.3a

Fig. 28.3b

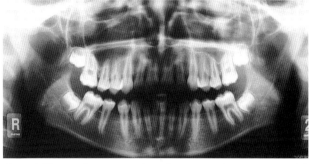

Fig. 28.3b Another case: dental panoramic tomogram (a) before and (b) following removal of all first permanent molars.

Key point

- Ensure all permanent teeth, especially 5's and 8's, are present radiographically before considering FPM extraction.
- Timing of extraction of $\bar{6}$ is more critical than that of 6̲.
- Consider balancing and/or compensating for extraction of a FPM.

What are the treatment options for the incisors in this case?

Microabrasion.

Localized composite restoration.

Full composite veneer.

Controlled enamel microabrasion may produce a more acceptable result without removing the white areas. This is because the surface enamel layer after microabrasion is relatively prismless and well compacted. The optical properties are changed and a white area may become less perceptible. The technique should not be used if there is a reduced thickness of enamel.

Localized composites can give very acceptable results but are destructive of enamel and may weaken the tooth structure if large areas are removed.

Full composite veneers with a thin layer of a relatively opaque composite may produce an acceptable result without any or very little enamel reduction.

Recommended reading

Beentjes VEVM, Weerheijm KL, Groen HI 2002 Factors involved in the aetiology of molar–incisor hypomineralisation (MIH). Eur J Paediatr Dent 1:9–13.

Jalevik B, Klingberg GA 2002 Dental treatment, dental fear and behaviour management problems in children with severe enamel hypomineralisation of their permanent first molars. Int J Paediatr Dent 12:24–32.

Mackie IC, Blinkhorn AS, Davies PHJ 1989 The extraction of permanent first molars during the mixed dentition period—a guide to treatment planning. J Paed Dent 5:85–92.

Zagdwon, AM, Toumba, KJ, Curzon, MEJ 2002 The prevalence of developmental defects in permanent molars in a group of English schoolchildren. Eur J Paediatr Dent 3:91–96.

29

Tooth discolouration, hypomineralization and hypoplasia

Case 1
Summary

Simon is 8. He has been brought to your surgery by his mother because his teeth are very dark and he is being teased at school. How would you determine the origin of the discolouration?

History

Simon says that the colour of his permanent teeth has remained the same since they erupted (**Fig. 29.1**).

What other questions do you need to ask about the teeth?

- Do they chip or wear?
- Was the primary dentition affected?
- Has anyone else in the family got, or had, similar teeth?

Positive answers to these questions may suggest an inherited abnormality of the teeth such as amelogenesis or dentinogenesis imperfecta.

Have you also noticed that he has gingival overgrowth?

Medical history

What specific questions do you need to ask his mother with regard to potential causes of discolouration?

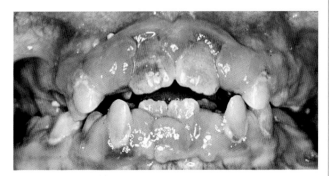

Fig. 29.1 Intrinsic discolouration.

• The pregnancy

The health of Simon's mother during her pregnancy and Simon's health during the birth and delivery are important when considering the condition of the first permanent molars (FPMs). The FPMs were the only permanent teeth that had started to mineralize before birth (≈ eighth month of pregnancy). Conditions that may suggest some fetal distress and dysmineralization may be: raised maternal blood pressure; early admission to hospital; premature delivery; prolonged delivery; assisted delivery, e.g. forceps or ventouse; emergency caesarean section; admission to the special care baby unit (SCBU).

• Childhood illnesses

These may result in a 'chronological hypoplasia' affecting those parts of the teeth that were mineralizing at the time of the illness. Although 'chronological hypoplasia' usually involves some failure of development of enamel matrix giving obvious lines or ridges on the teeth, there may be milder forms that can only be felt with a probe and that present for care because they attract extrinsic stain.

• Tablets or medications taken during childhood

Tetracycline staining should not occur now in children who have been brought up in developed countries. It is still common in children from developing countries where tetracycline is still used because it is a very effective, cheap, broadspectrum antibiotic. The only children who may still be affected in developed countries are those with cystic fibrosis who have developed muliple drug resistances as a result of recurrent respiratory infection.

Simon was born with primary biliary atresia. This resulted in progressive liver failure, increasing levels of circulating bilirubin and eventually a liver transplant at the age of 2.5 years. All the permanent teeth developing prior to the transplantation will have intrinsic discolouration as a result of the high circulating bilirubin. The primary dentition will be affected to a lesser extent as a result of staining in secondary dentine. He has gingival overgrowth as a result of immunosuppressive treatment with cyclosporin. **Figure 29.2** shows a photograph taken at the age of 13. The newly erupted second permanent molars are entirely normal. These teeth started mineralizing about the age of 3 when there was a functioning new liver and normal levels of bilirubin.

• Dental history
What other lines of questioning do we need to explore if we are considering all the possible causes of intrinsic discolouration?

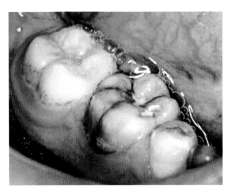

Fig. 29.2 Normal colour of second permanent molar.

Was there a history of infection and/or extraction for decay of any of the primary teeth?

Localized infection on primary teeth can cause localized abnormalities of enamel formation and mineralization of permanent teeth.

Was there ever any trauma to the primary teeth?

There is a 50% chance of enamel dysmineralization of permanent successor teeth after primary trauma. These will be localized anomalies.

Fluoride history

A full history from birth including areas that the child has lived in, fluoride supplementation and brushing habits is required. Fluorosis will produce a systemic or chronological distribution affecting the teeth that were forming when excess fluoride was taken.

The important categories and questions for a history into intrinsic tooth discolouration and hypoplasia are shown in **Box 29.1**.

Examination

The important features to note about any intrinsic discolouration or hypoplasia are:

Is it generalized or localized?

Does it affect the primary and permanent dentitions?

In the major categories for questioning shown in Box 29.1, which are likely to cause generalized discolouration and which are likely to cause localized discolouration?

Generalized: medical; family; fluorosis.

Localized: pregnancy; dental; trauma.

Simon has generalized intrinsic discolouration as a result of biliary atresia causing increased levels of bilirubin.

What is the only method of treatment that will help Simon's appearance?

Veneering. Composite veneers should be provided until the age of 16 years when they can be replaced with

---

Box 29.1 Intrinsic tooth discolouration and hypoplasia

Maternal and neonatal history
- History of pregnancy—maternal problems
- History of birth—caesarean, forceps, fetal distress

Family history
- Is anyone in the family similarly affected

Medical history
- Dates of prolonged illnesses, e.g. the childhood infections, haematological disorders, nutritional diseases etc.
- Medications taken

Dental history
- Does the discolouration affect all the teeth or just a few teeth
- Does the discolouration affect both primary and permanent dentitions
- Has it got worse or did the teeth come through like it
- History of abscesses of the primary dentition
- Any pain from teeth
- Are the teeth chipping or wearing away

Trauma history
- Has the child any history of an accident to primary or permanent teeth

Fluoride history
- Where has the child lived
- History of fluoride supplements
- Age at commencement of brushing
- Amount and type of toothpaste
- Toothpaste eating

---

porcelain veneers. Composite veneers may not mask the severe green stain unless opaquing agents are used. Porcelain veneers may be the only realistic alternative and can be provided at a younger age by using a smaller amount of enamel reduction and accepting a slightly thicker final tooth size.

The method of placement of composite veneers is covered in Chapter 30.

Key point

Lines of questioning in discolouration, hypomineralization and hypoplasia:
- Maternal.
- Trauma.
- Medical.
- Fluoride.
- Dental.
- Family.

If a patient came to you with a single discoloured root-filled incisor what form of treatment should you consider first?

Non-vital bleaching. This technique has certain advantages, especially in the younger and adolescent patient:

Non-destructive of tooth tissue (already root filled).

No irritation to gingival health that can occur with veneers.

No change in contour of tooth that may make oral hygiene more difficult.

No laboratory assistance required.

The only contraindications to non-vital bleaching would be teeth that already have large composite restorations, teeth that have been stained due to placement of amalgam into an access cavity and poorly obturated teeth.

There are a number of bleaching products available now that can be applied intracoronally. Most of these will contain hydrogen peroxide. However, bleaching can be achieved with sodium perborate alone as the following technique describes.

● Materials

1. Rubber dam.
2. Zinc phosphate cement.
3. 37% phosphoric acid.
4. Sodium perborate (Bocasan) powder: distilled water.
5. Cotton wool.
6. Glass ionomer cement.
7. White gutta percha.
8. Composite resin.

● Technique

1. Take preoperative periapical radiographs; these are essential to check there is an adequate root filling.
2. Clean the teeth with pumice and make a note of the shade of the discoloured tooth.
3. Place rubber dam, isolating the single tooth. Ensure adequate eye protection for the patient, operator and dental nurse.
4. Remove palatal restoration and pulp chamber restoration.
5. Remove root filling to the level of the dentogingival junction—you may need to use adult burs in a miniature contra-angle head.
6. Place 1 mm of zinc phosphate or glass ionomer cement (GIC) over the gutta percha.
7. Freshen dentine with a round bur. Do not remove excessively.
8. Etch the pulp chamber with 37% phosphoric acid for 30–60 seconds, wash and dry—this will facilitate the ingress of the bleach.
9. Mix the sodium perborate into a thick paste. This should be done immediately before placement. Place into the tooth, either alone with a flat plastic instrument or on a cotton-wool pledget.
10. Place a dry piece of cotton wool over the perborate mixture.
11. Seal the cavity with glass ionomer cement or intermediate restorative material cement.
12. Repeat the process at weekly intervals until the tooth is slightly overbleached.
13. Place non-setting calcium hydroxide into the pulp chamber for 2 weeks. Seal with GIC.
14. Finally, restore the tooth with white gutta percha (to facilitate reopening the pulp chamber again, if necessary, at a later date) and composite resin.

If the colour of a tooth has not significantly improved after three changes of bleach then it is unlikely to do so, and further bleaching should be abandoned. Failure of a tooth to bleach could be due to inadequate removal of filling materials from the pulp chamber.

Slight overbleaching is desirable, but the patient should be instructed to attend the surgery before the next appointment if marked overbleaching has occurred.

Non-vital bleaching has a reputation of causing brittleness of the tooth. This is probably the result of previous injudicious removal of dentine (which only needs to be 'freshened' with a round bur), rather than a direct effect of the bleaching procedure itself.

This method of bleaching has been associated with the later occurrence of external cervical resorption. The exact mechanism of this association is unclear, but it is thought that the bleach diffuses through the dentinal tubules to set up an inflammatory reaction in the periodontal ligament around the cervical region of the tooth. In a small number of teeth there is a gap between enamel and cementum, and in these cases the above explanation is tenable. The purpose of the 1-mm layer of cement is to cover the openings of the dentinal tubules at the level where there may be a communication to the periodontal ligament. In the same way, non-setting calcium hydroxide is placed in the pulp chamber for 2 weeks prior to final restoration in order to eradicate any inflammation in the periodontal ligament that may have been initiated.

Clinical studies have demonstrated that regression can be expected with this technique. The longest study after 8 years gave a 21% failure rate. However, if white gutta percha has been placed within the pulp chamber then it is readily removed and the tooth easily rebleached.

Key point

Restorative techniques in discolouration
● Microabrasion.
● Bleaching.
● Localized composite.
● Veneers.

Case 2
Summary

Tony is 14. He has come to your surgery because he is concerned by the colour of his teeth and his bad breath (Fig. 29.3).

History

He has noticed his teeth changing colour over the past year. His friends have also commented on his bad breath over this period of time.

The colour of the teeth in **Figure 29.3** is a result of extrinsic staining from chromogenic bacteria due to inadequate oral hygiene. The staining is classically in the gingival and cervical areas of the teeth.

Are there any other causes of extrinsic staining?

Food and drink. Tea, coffee and dishes such as curry can cause staining of the teeth. Most commonly this occurs in the gingival or cervical areas initially, but if oral hygiene is poor then it can affect a significant part of the whole tooth surface (**Fig. 29.4**).

Arrested caries. This produces a brown stain as a result of chromogenic bacteria.

Medical condition. In biliary atresia and jaundice it is possible for bile pigments in the gingival crevicular fluid to cause extrinsic staining. This is yellow/green in colour.

Drugs. Ferrous sulphate in liquid iron preparations can result in black staining. Rifabutin, an antituberculous drug, is excreted in the crevicular fluid. This results in an orange-red staining.

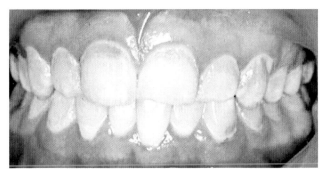

Fig. 29.3 Extrinsic chromogenic staining.

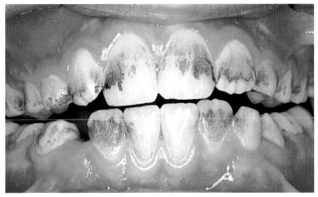

Fig. 29.4 Extrinsic food staining.

Chlorhexidine mouthwash when used frequently can cause a brown-black staining.

All these extrinsic stains originate initially around the gingival or cervical area of the tooth but can progress to involve a significant amount of the tooth surface.

How can you confirm your diagnosis of extrinsic discolouration?

Extrinsic stains can be polished off. Carry out a prophylaxis.

What additional clinical signs are there on Figure 29.3 to back up your diagnosis of chromogenic staining secondary to poor oral hygiene?

Marginal gingivitis.

'White spot' demineralization lesions in the gingival third of the labial enamel are visible on the anterior teeth.

Treatment
How would you treat Tony's bad breath?

Encourage him. Remember teenagers don't take criticism well! Tell him that he is not alone and lots of 'busy' young people forget twice daily brushing.

Toothbrushing instruction utilizing disclosing tablets or disclosing solution. Brushing twice daily, after breakfast and before school, and then last thing at night with a 1000–1500 ppm paste.

Show him the 'white spot' lesions. Explain that these will progress to decay if the brushing is not corrected.

Daily fluoride mouthwash 0.05% sodium fluoride to encourage enamel remineralization.

What factors in children and adolescents are important in halitosis (bad breath)?

Plaque index.

Bleeding sites in gingiva.

Food impaction.

Nasal infection.

Tonsillar and adenoidal infection.

Furred tongue especially posterior tongue.

As well as improving his gingival health with improved toothbrushing, what else could be done with the toothbrush?

Brushing the dorsum of his tongue! Alternative methods can be used to clean the surface of the tongue and various types of 'tongue scrapers' are available commercially. Very occasionally in a child or adolescent the origin of halitosis can be ulceration of oesophageal or gastric origin. If there are symptoms of this then a referral should be made.

Recommended reading

Kilpatrick NM, Welbury RR 2001 Advanced restorative dentistry. In: Welbury RR (ed) Paediatric dentistry, 2nd edn.Oxford University Press, Oxford.

Wray A, Welbury RR 2001 UK national guidelines in paediatric dentistry: treatment of intrinsic discolouration in permanent anterior teeth in children and adolescents. Int J Paediatr Dent 11:309–315.

For revision see Mind Map 29, page 175

30

Mottled teeth

Summary

Sophie is 8. Her main concern is that all her permanent teeth have white patches, especially the upper central incisors. She is getting teased at school because the upper centrals also have brown patches. What are the causes of the white patches? How may they be treated?

History

Sophie noticed that the permanent teeth came through with the white and brown patches (**Fig. 30.1**). They have not changed in appearance since eruption.

What important questions would you now ask her mother?

Were the primary teeth normal?

If the answer to this is yes then it is unlikely to be an inherited defect and more likely to have a systemic origin.

Is anyone else in the family affected?

Unless siblings are subjected to exactly the same systemic diseases and conditions it is likely that an affected sibling will indicate an inherited defect.

Sophie's primary teeth were normal and she had no siblings, but neither her mother's nor her father's family had anyone with a similar problem.

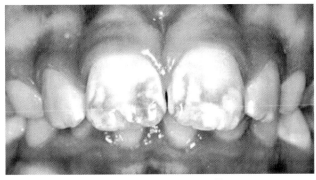

Fig. 30.1 Disfiguring fluorotic mottling affecting upper permanent central incisors.

What childhood illnesses and infections did she have, and when?

A chronological hypomineralization or hypoplasia would suggest a systemic origin. There were no significant illnesses.

What is Sophie's fluoride history?

This must include where she has lived, any history of supplements, type of toothpaste used, amount of toothpaste used, any history of eating toothpaste.

It transpired that Sophie had never received any supplements, nor used toothpaste excessively. However, she lived on a farm with its own 'well' water supply. This was subsequently analysed and was found to be over 1 ppm fluoride. The diagnosis was one of fluorosis.

What is the distribution of the mottling that you can see in Figure 30.1?

White and brown mottling of the incisal half of the labial surface of 1|1 and white mottling of the incisal third of the labial surface of 2|2 .

Do you know why the labial surfaces of the upper permanent central incisors are often more affected by mottling?

Research has shown that these teeth are particularly susceptible to an excess ingestion of fluoride between 24 and 30 months of age.

Mild fluorosis gives a diffuse mottling that may manifest as diffuse lines or patches that merge into the background enamel. When the fluorosis becomes more severe the lines and patches coalesce to produce a confluent white surface. In very severe cases there is also pitting of the enamel. Well-defined or well-demarcated patches that do not follow a systemic or chronological distribution, or are localized, are not likely to be due to fluorosis.

Which part of the enamel does mild fluorosis affect?

The outer 200–300 µm.

How can you use this knowledge to your advantage during your clinical examination?

Look for areas of the dentition that are subject to erosion or attrition, e.g. the occlusal surfaces of the first permanent molars. If the mottled enamel has been removed on these surfaces then that confirms that the mottling is

> ### Key point
>
> History taking in suspected fluorosis:
> - Fluoridated water in places of residence.
> - Amount of paste and age brushing started.
> - Supplements.
> - 'Eating' toothpaste.

in the outer aspect of the enamel and the diagnosis is likely to be one of fluorosis.

In some cases of fluorosis there is, in addition to white mottling, some brown stain. What is the cause of the brown staining?

This is usually due to extrinsic agents becoming incorporated into the more porous white mottled areas of enamel. The brown mottling tends to get worse with time.

What treatment options for Sophie would you consider for fluorotic mottling?

Microabrasion.

Composite veneers.

Microabrasion can be done in a variety of ways and is a controlled removal of the surface layer of enamel in order to improve discolourations that are limited to the outer enamel layer. It is not suitable for deep enamel or dentine discolouration. One of the most reliable methods that has been used extensively since 1986 is the hydrochloric acid–pumice microabrasion technique. It is achieved by a combination of abrasion and erosion—the term 'abrosion' is sometimes used. In the clinical technique that will be described, no more than 100 µm of enamel is removed. Once completed the procedure should not be repeated again in the future. Too much enamel removal is potentially damaging to the pulp and cosmetically the underlying dentine colour will become more evident.

Indications:

1. Fluorosis.
2. Idiopathic speckling.
3. Postorthodontic treatment demineralization.
4. Prior to veneer placement for well-demarcated stains.
5. White/brown surface staining, e.g. secondary to primary predecessor infection or trauma (Turner teeth).

Materials:

1. Bicarbonate of soda/water.
2. Copalite varnish/Vaseline.
3. Fluoridated toothpaste.
4. Non-acidulated fluoride (fluoride drops).
5. Pumice.
6. Rubber dam.
7. Rubber prophylaxis cup.
8. Soflex polishing discs.
9. 18% hydrochloric acid.

Technique:

1. Perform preoperative vitality tests, take radiographs and photographs.
2. Clean the teeth with pumice and water, wash and dry.
3. Isolate the teeth to be treated with rubber dam, and paint Copalite varnish around the necks of the dam (alternatively place Vaseline around the necks of the teeth under the rubber dam).
4. Place a mixture of sodium bicarbonate and water on the dam behind the teeth, as protection in case of spillage.
5. Mix 18% hydrochloric acid with pumice into a slurry and apply a small amount to the labial surface on either a rubber prophylaxis cup rotating slowly or a wooden stick rubbed over the surface for 5 seconds, before washing for 5 seconds directly into an aspirator tip. Repeat until the stain is reduced, up to a maximum of 10×5 seconds applications per tooth. Any improvement that is going to occur will have done so by this time.
6. Apply the fluoride drops to the teeth for 3 minutes.
7. Remove the rubber dam.
8. Polish the teeth with the finest Soflex discs.
9. Polish the teeth with fluoridated toothpaste for 1 minute.
10. Review in 1 month for vitality tests and clinical photographs (**Fig. 30.2**).
11. Review biannually, checking pulpal status.

Critical analysis of the effectiveness of the technique should not be made immediately but delayed for at least 1 month as the appearance of the teeth will continue to improve over this time. Experience has shown that brown mottling is removed more easily than white, but even where white mottling is incompletely removed it nevertheless becomes less perceptible. This phenomenon has been attributed to the relatively prismless layer of compacted surface enamel produced by the 'abrosion' technique, which alters the optical properties of the tooth surface.

Long-term studies of the technique have found no association with pulpal damage, increased caries susceptibility or significant prolonged thermal sensitivity. Patient compliance and satisfaction is good and any dissatisfaction is usually due to inadequate preoperative explanation. The technique is easy to perform for the operator and patient, and is not time-consuming. Removal of any mottled area is permanent and achieved with an insignificant loss of surface enamel. Failure to improve appearance by the HCl–pumice microabrasion technique has no harmful effects but may make it easier to mask some lesions with veneers.

Key point

Microabrasion:
- Will improve surface defects, e.g. fluorosis.
- Will not improve deeper defects, e.g. amelogenesis imperfecta.

Figure 30.2 shows the appearance of Sophie's 1|1 1 month after HCl–pumice microabrasion.

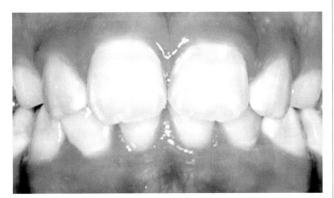

Fig. 30.2 After acid pumice microabrasion.

Has bleaching of teeth any part to play in the treatment of surface enamel discolouration?

Yes, external vital bleaching has been used as an initial treatment for fluorotic mottling and as a secondary treatment for residual brown staining after microabrasion. It is, however, more usually associated with the bleaching of the yellow discolouration of ageing—so-called 'nightguard vital bleaching'. This technique involves the daily placement of carbamide peroxide gel into a custom-fitted tray of either the upper or the lower arch. As the name suggests it is carried out by the patient at home and is initially done on a daily basis.

Materials:
1. Upper impression and working model.
2. Soft mouthguard—avoiding the gingivae.
3. 10% carbamide peroxide gel.

Technique:
1. Take an alginate impression of the arch to be treated and cast a working model in stone.
2. Relieve the labial surfaces of the teeth by about 0.5 mm and make a soft, pull-down, vacuum-formed splint as a mouthguard. The splint should be no more than 2 mm in thickness and should not cover the gingivae. It is only a vehicle for the bleaching gel and not intended to protect the gingivae.
3. Instruct the patient on how to floss the teeth thoroughly. Perform a full mouth prophylaxis and instruct them how to apply the gel into the mouthguard.
4. Note that the length of time the guard should be worn depends on the product used.
5. Review about 2 weeks later to check that the patient is not experiencing any sensitivity, and then at 6 weeks, by which time 80% of any colour change should have occurred.

Carbamide peroxide gel (10%) breaks down in the mouth into 3% hydrogen peroxide and 7% urea. Both urea and hydrogen peroxide have low molecular weights, which allow them to diffuse rapidly through enamel and dentine and thus explains the transient pulpal sensitivity occasionally experienced with home bleaching systems.

Pulpal histology with regard to these materials has not been assessed, but no clinical significance has been attributed to the changes seen with 35% hydrogen peroxide over 75 years of usage, except where teeth have been overheated or traumatized. By extrapolation, 3% hydrogen peroxide in the home systems should therefore be safe.

Although most carbamide peroxide materials contain trace amounts of phosphoric and citric acids as stabilizers and preservatives, no indication of etching or a significant change in the surface morphology of enamel has been demonstrated by scanning electron microscopy analysis. There was early concern that bleaching solutions with a low pH would cause demineralization of enamel when the pH fell below the 'critical' pH of 5.2–5.8. However, no evidence of this process has been noted to date in any clinical trials or laboratory tests, and this may be due to the urea (and subsequently the ammonia) and carbon dioxide released on degradation of the carbamide peroxide elevating the pH.

There is an initial decrease in bond strength of enamel to composite resin immediately after home bleaching but this returns to normal within 7 days. This effect has been attributed to the residual oxygen in the bleached tooth surface, which inhibits polymerization of the composite resin. The home bleaching systems do not affect the colour of restorative materials. Any perceived effect is probably due to superficial cleansing.

Minor ulceration or irritation may occur during the initial treatment. It is important to check that the mouthguard does not extend on to the gingivae and that the edges of the guard are smooth. If ulceration persists a decreased exposure time may be necessary. If there is still a problem then allergy is a possibility.

The exact mechanism of bleaching is unknown. Theories of oxidation, photo-oxidation and ion exchange have been suggested. Conversely, the cause of rediscolouration is also unknown. This may be a combination of chemical reduction of the oxidation products previously formed, marginal leakage of restorations allowing ingress of bacterial and chemical byproducts, and salivary or tissue fluid contamination via permeable tooth structure.

Dense fluorotic white plaques and some forms of hypomature amelogenesis imperfecta may be clinically indistinguishable. The microabrasion technique in this situation can be used as a diagnostic aid. Improvement in appearance would support the diagnosis of fluorosis, which affects the outer layer of enamel, whereas amelogenesis commonly affects the whole enamel layer.

Composite veneers may be required to mask dense white fluorotic plaques that are refractory to microabrasion. Most composite veneers placed in children and adolescents are the direct type fashioned at the chairside rather than the indirect or laboratory-made type.

Before proceeding with any veneering technique, the decision must be made whether to reduce the thickness of labial enamel before placing the veneer. Certain factors should be considered:

1. Increased labiopalatal bulk makes it harder to maintain good oral hygiene. This may be courting disaster in the adolescent with a dubious oral hygiene technique.
2. Composite resin has a better bond strength to enamel when the surface layer of 200–300 μm is removed.
3. If a tooth is very discoloured some sort of reduction will be desirable, as a thicker layer of composite will be required to mask the intense stain.
4. If a tooth is already instanding or rotated, its appearance can be enhanced by a thicker labial veneer.

New generation, highly polishable, hybrid composite resins can replace relatively large amounts of missing tooth tissue as well as being used in thin sections as a veneer. Combinations of shades can be used to simulate natural colour gradations and hues.

Indications for composite veneers:
1. Discolouration.
2. Enamel defects.
3. Diastemata.
4. Malpositioned teeth.
5. Large restorations.

Contraindications:
1. Insufficient available enamel for bonding.
2. Oral habits, e.g. woodwind musicians.

Materials:
1. Rubber dam/contoured matrix strips (Vivadent).
2. Preparation and finishing burs.
3. New generation, highly polishable, hybrid composite resin.
4. Soflex polishing discs and interproximal polishing strips.

Technique:
1. Use a tapered diamond bur to reduce labial enamel by 0.3–0.5 mm. Identify the finish line at the gingival margin and also mesially and distally just labial to the contact points.
2. Clean the tooth with a slurry of pumice in water. Wash and dry and select the shade.

3. Isolate the tooth either with rubber dam or a contoured matrix strip. Hold the latter in place by applying unfilled resin to its gingival side against the gingiva and curing for 10 seconds.
4. Etch the enamel for 60 seconds, wash and dry.
5. Where dentine is exposed apply dentine primer.
6. Apply a thin layer of bonding resin to the labial surface and roughly shape it into all areas with a plastic instrument, then use a brush lubricated with unfilled resin to 'paddle' and smooth it into the desired shape. Cure for 60 seconds gingivally, 60 seconds mesio-incisally, 60 seconds disto-incisally, and 60 seconds from the palatal aspect if incisal coverage has been used. Different shades of composite can be combined to achieve good matches with adjacent teeth and a transition from a relatively dark gingival area to a lighter more translucent incisal region.
8. Flick away the unfilled resin holding the contour strip and remove the strip.
9. Finish the margins with diamond finishing burs and interproximal strips and the labial surface with graded sandpaper discs. Characterization should be added to improve light reflection properties.

The exact design of the composite veneer will be dependent upon each clinical case, but will usually be one of four types: intraenamel or window preparation; incisal bevel; overlapped incisal edge; or feathered incisal edge.

Tooth preparation will not normally expose dentine, but this will be unavoidable in some cases of localized hypoplasia or with caries. Sound dentine may need to be covered by glass ionomer cement prior to placement of the composite veneer.

Recommended reading

Croll TP, Cavanaugh RR 1986 Enamel colour modification by controlled hydrochloric acid-pumice abrasion. I. Technique and examples. Quintessence Int 17:81–87.

Heywood VB, Heymann HO 1989 Nightguard vital bleaching. Quintessence Int 20:173–176.

Kilpatrick NM, Welbury RR. Advanced restorative dentistry. In: Welbury RR (ed) Paediatric dentistry, 2nd edn. Oxford University Press, Oxford, pp 189–215.

For revision see Mind Map 30, page 176

31
Tooth surface loss

Summary

Tom is 9. He is a new patient to your practice. On examination you are concerned by the appearance of the occlusal surfaces of his lower primary molars. What has caused this and how may it be managed?

What do you see (Fig. 31.1)?

There is erosion of the cusps of his primary molars giving cupping or perimolysis of the cusps with loss of enamel and visible underlying dentine.

How would you define erosion?

An irreversible loss of tooth substance brought about by a chemical process that does not involve bacterial action.

What foods and drinks have erosive potential?

See **Box 31.1**. While a wide range of food and drinks is implicated in the problem, the bulk of the damage is done by soft drinks, especially carbonated drinks, which are increasingly available from vending machines in schools and recreational facilities. All carbonated drinks and fruit-based drinks have lowered pH values but the direct relationship between pH and erosion is unclear. Other factors such as titratable acidity, the influence of plaque

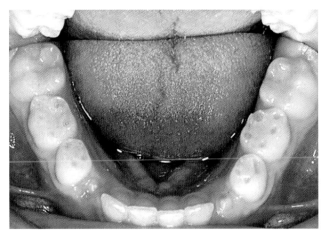

Fig. 31.1 Erosion of cusp tips of primary molars.

Box 31.1 Erosive potential of foods and drinks

- Citrus fruits, e.g. lemons, oranges, grapefruits
- Tart apples
- Vinegar and pickles
- Yoghurt
- All fruit juices including fresh juice and fruit-based squashes
- Carbonated drinks, including low calorie varieties, 'sports drinks' and sparkling mineral water
- Vitamin C tablets

pH and the buffering capacity of saliva will all influence the erosive potential of a substrate. Three things, however, are clear with erosive loss:

> It is worse if consumption is high.
> It is worse if consumption occurs at bedtime.
> It is worse if brushing occurs directly after consumption.

History

Tom's only complaint was occasional sensitivity on his back teeth as a result of the visible dentine.

What is the best way to find out about Tom's diet?

A 3- or 4-day written dietary history is the only way to accurately elucidate a constituent of the diet that may be erosive.

Can the pattern of erosion caused by dietary constituents be related to the manner in which the substrate is consumed?

This is indeed the case. 'Frothing' of a drink between the upper anterior teeth with its retention labially can lead to palatal, interproximal and labial erosion. Retention of a drink specifically on one side of the mouth can lead to erosion on that side only.

You have covered Tom's dietary history. Is your history now complete or are there other questions you need to ask with relation to erosion?

It is very important to consider gastric acid as a cause of erosion, even in a younger patient. The conditions in children that are associated with chronic regurgitation are shown in **Box 31.2**. The acidity of the stomach contents is below pH 1.0 and therefore any regurgitation or vomiting is damaging to the teeth.

What question would you ask to give you an indication that regurgitation was occurring?

'Do you ever have a bitter taste in your mouth?' There is a group of patients who suffer from gastro-oesophageal reflux disease (GORD). This may be either symptomatic,

---

Box 31.2 Conditions associated with chronic regurgitation in children

Gastro-oesophageal reflux
Oesophageal stricture
Chronic respiratory disease, e.g. asthma
Disease of the liver/pancreas/biliary tree
Overfeeding
Feeding problems/failure to thrive conditions
Mental handicap
Cerebral palsy
Rumination

---

in which the individual knows what provokes the reflux, or more insidiously, asymptomatic GORD, where the patient is unaware of the problem. The latter case is most likely to occur at night when the horizontal sleeping position makes it more likely that acid will reflux through the lower oesophageal sphincter. In this case the question about a bitter taste in the mouth should have the suffix 'when you wake up'.

What is the common pattern of erosive loss when there is chronic gastric regurgitation?

Initially there is erosion of the palatal surfaces of the upper incisors, canines and premolars. With time this extends to the occlusal and buccal surfaces of the lower molars and premolars.

Whenever there is unexplained erosive loss, an eating disorder should be suspected. There are three such disorders: anorexia nervosa; bulimia nervosa; rumination. The latter is a condition in which food is voluntarily regurgitated into the oral cavity and either expelled or swallowed again.

Is there a specific pattern of erosive loss in recurrent vomiting?

All tooth surfaces can be affected with the relative exception of the lingual surfaces of the lower teeth, which are protected by the tongue and the saliva from the sublingual papillae.

What would you do if you suspect after questioning Tom and his parents that there may be asymptomatic GORD?

Referral to a paediatrician with an interest in gastro-intestinal disease would be appropriate. The paediatrician will seek to eliminate organic disease and then attempt to quantify the problem. The latter may involve 24-hour pH monitoring of the oesophagus with probes in the lower and upper oesophagus. An additional probe could be added to an intraoral appliance to measure mouth pH. Medical and/or surgical treatment may be required to control GORD. Chronic regurgitation can lead to scarring of the oesophagus and dysplastic change, and this is therefore an important condition to diagnose and treat.

• Summary of Tom's history

There was no evidence of any gastrointestinal illness but Tom did consume a number of fizzy drinks, especially between meals and when he was at the local sports centre. In addition to these he also drank water and milk.

What advice would you give to Tom regarding his high intake of fizzy drinks?

It is critically important when dealing with children and adolescents not to be too dogmatic in your advice.

It is unrealistic to expect youngsters who have been brought up with a high intake of carbonated beverages to stop altogether. They should be advised to eradicate between-meal fizzy drink consumption but to have the fizzy drink with meals and preferably to drink it with a straw. The presence of food, and the extra saliva that is generated at mealtimes, will help to neutralize the acidity. In addition, a straw will deposit the majority of the carbonated beverage beyond the teeth.

Make sure that the between-meal carbonated drink is not substituted by something with a similar erosive potential, e.g. fresh fruit juice or a juice-based squash.

Milk and water are the most appropriate between-meal drinks. If either of these proves impossible then an extremely well diluted 'no added sugar' squash can be accepted.

No carbonated drinks or fruit drinks should be given last thing at night.

Advocate the consumption of a neutral food imme-diately after a meal, e.g. cheese.

Management

The most important aspect of the management of Tom's erosion was early diagnosis before there had been damage to the permanent teeth, and subsequently to establish the aetiology and eliminate the cause.

Key point

Management of erosion:
● Early diagnosis.
● Establish aetiology.
● Eliminate cause.

Tom only has occasional sensitivity. What treatment, if any, does he need?

Probably none. The following would be realistic initially:
Daily neutral sodium fluoride mouthwash to try and give maximum resistance to remaining enamel and desensitize dentine
High concentration sodium fluoride varnish (Duraphat) to be applied three times a year.
If there is progressive sensitivity then the areas of enamel loss and dentine exposure could be protected by an adhesive

restoration. In many cases if erosion is diagnosed early then preventive counselling and the above advice may be sufficient. It is a good idea to make study casts of all patients with signs of erosion or attrition or abrasion to monitor the rate of progression. In more advanced cases than Tom, as in **Figures 31.2a** and **b** where there is significant sensitivity or cosmetic problems, then more active intervention is required. **Table 31.1** shows the merits of the different options available.

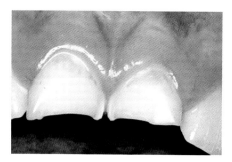

Fig. 31.2 a

Fig. 31.2 b

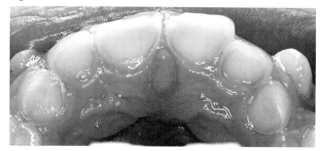

Fig. 31.2 (a,b) Significant erosive tooth surface loss of labial and palatal surfaces of upper permanent incisors.

Key point

Treatment objectives for erosion:
● Resolve sensitivity.
● Restore missing tooth surface.
● Prevent further tooth tissue loss.
● Maintain a balanced occlusion.

Erosion is only one element of tooth surface loss or wear. What are the other elements?

Attrition: the wear of the tooth as a result of tooth-to-tooth contact.

Abrasion: physical wear of tooth substance produced by something other than tooth-to-tooth contact.

In children, abrasion is usually due to overzealous toothbrushing, which tends to develop with increasing age. The abnormal brushing technique must be corrected before significant tooth tissue is removed and pulpal exposure occurs. Attrition caused by normal mastication is common especially with the ageing primary dentition. Almost all primary teeth show signs of attrition by the time they exfoliate.

What categories of patient exhibit more attrition than normal?

Those with significant parafunctional activity, e.g. cerebral palsy and other physical and developmental disorders with intracranial abnormalities. Controlling attritional wear in these patients can be very difficult. Some drugs act to try to reduce such parafunctional activity but even if this is successful in the limbs there is often still residual oral parafunction. This is probably due to the neuronal sensitivity of the mouth and the structures within it.

Table 31.1 Treatment techniques for tooth surface loss

Technique	Advantages	Disadvantages
Cast metal (nickel/chrome or gold)	Fabricated in thin section—requires only 0.5-mm space Very accurate fit possible Very durable Suitable for posterior restorations in parafunction Does not abrade opposing dentition	May be cosmetically unacceptable due to 'shine through' of metallic grey Cannot be simply repaired or added to intraorally
Composite: direct	Least expensive Can be added to and repaired intraorally Aesthetically superior to cast metal	Technically difficult for palatal veneers Limited control over occlusal and interproximal contour Inadequate as a posterior restoration
Composite: indirect	Can be added to and repaired intraorally Aesthetically superior to cast metal Control over occlusal contour and vertical dimension	Requires more space—minimum of 1.0 mm. Unproven durability
Porcelain	Best aesthetics Good abrasion resistance Well tolerated by gingival tissues	Potentially abrasive to opposing dentition Inferior marginal fit Very brittle—has to be used in bulk section Hard to repair

What restorative materials are the most durable for attritional wear as a result of parafunction?

Amalgam and stainless steel crowns.

Recommended reading

Kilpatrick, NM, Welbury RR 2001 Advanced restorative dentistry. In: Welbury RR (ed) Paediatric dentistry, 2nd edn. Oxford University Press, Oxford, pp 189–215.

Shaw L, O'Sullivan E 2000 UK National Clinical Guidelines in Paediatric Dentistry. Diagnosis and prevention of dental erosion in children. Int J Paediatr Dent 10:356–365.

For revision see Mind Map 3, page 177

32

Multiple missing and abnormally shaped teeth

Case 1
Summary

Ellen is almost 11. She is very concerned by the gaps between her upper and lower front teeth. She is hoping to become an actress. She is a new patient to your surgery and has been brought by her mother. What are the causes of the problem and how may it be treated?

History

Ellen is a regular attender with no caries. Her oral hygiene is excellent. There is no history of tooth extraction of either the primary or permanent dentitions.

● Medical history

Ellen has no medical problems. She is an active girl who is involved in orienteering with her family as well as being in the local amateur dramatic society.

What question do you need to ask Ellen's mother?

Is there a family history of missing teeth or gaps?

As you are speaking to Ellen's mother you notice that she has a missing upper right lateral incisor with the canine tooth prominent. She confirms your question that not only has she got a missing tooth, but her brother and her nephew (son of her brother) have either missing or very small upper lateral incisors.

How prevalent are missing teeth in the population?

0.1–0.9% in the primary dentition.
3.5–6.5% in the permanent dentition (discounting third molars).
More common in females, than males (1.4–4×).

The most common teeth to be absent are the last teeth in each series (i.e. lateral incisor, second premolar, third molar). The presence of a conical (peg) tooth is frequently associated with a missing tooth on the opposite side of the arch. There is frequently a family history.

There are a significant number of syndromes of the head and neck that manifest missing teeth. Can you name some?

Ectodermal dysplasia.
Cleft lip and/or palate.
Down syndrome.
Chondro-ectodermal dysplasia (Ellis–van Creveld syndrome).
Reiger's syndrome.
Incontinentia pigmenti.
Oro-facial-digital syndrome (Types I and II).

Ectodermal dysplasia describes a group of inherited disorders involving ectodermally derived structures, i.e. hair, teeth, nails, skin and sweat glands. The most common form is the hypohydrotic X-linked form. The usual presentation is a male child with:

Multiple congenital absence of teeth.
Fine, sparse hair with shaft abnormalities.
Dry skin.
Frontal bossing.
Maxillary hypoplasia.
Thin lips showing little vermilion margin.

Heterozygous females can be identified dentally with microdontia and hypodontia.

Down syndrome affects 1 in 700 births and is commoner in older mothers as a result of chromosomal translocation. Apart from the morphological features characteristic of the syndrome, there is commonly delayed eruption and generalized microdontia as well as hypodontia of some teeth.

The diagnosis and management of all dental anomalies is extremely important and should not be delayed. Genetic consultation is often desirable to not only confirm the diagnosis but also to help parents understand the risk of future offspring and generations being affected. Conversely, geneticists may require help from paediatric dentists to clarify a diagnosis.

Key point

Hypodontia:
● Is prevalent at 3.5–6.5% in permanent dentition (excepting third molar).
● May be associated with a number of syndromes.
● Requires multidisciplinary care.

What factors would you consider important in the management of dental anomalies?

Reassurance of child and parent.
Elimination of pain.
Genetic counselling.
Restoration of aesthetics.

Provision of adequate function.

Maintenance of vertical dimension of occlusion.

Interdisciplinary formulation of definitive treatment plan.

Examination

- Extra-oral

Ellen had a normal facial appearance with a Class 1 skeletal pattern.

- Intra-oral

The following teeth were present:

$$\frac{6\ e\ d\ c\ b\ 1\ |\ 1\ b\ c\ d\ e\ 6}{6\ a\quad 3\ 2\ 1\ |\quad 2\ 3\ 4\ e\ 6}$$

d|d were mobile. The other primary teeth were firm. The primary molars were infra-occluded.

What special investigations are required?

A dental panoramic tomogram (**Fig. 32.1**) to check on the present/absence of other permanent teeth.

What is visible from the radiograph?

Absence of: $\dfrac{8\ 7\ 5\ 3\ 2\ |\ 2\ 3\ 4\ 5\ 7\ 8}{8\ 7\ 5\ 4\ \ |\ 1\qquad\ 5\ 7}$

What is the condition known as?

It is termed severe hypodontia.

What would you do?

Take impressions and a wax registration for study models. Arrange a joint consultation with paediatric dental/ orthodontic/restorative colleagues.

What treatment is likely to be required?

- Attempt to retain the primary molars for as long as possible.
- Management of infra-occluded molars is dealt with in Chapter 6.
- Fixed appliance to close the upper median diastema; retain with a palatal bonded retainer
- Assess mesio-distal width 1|1. Probable addition of composite to distal aspect of these teeth to bring mesio-distal width to 8.5–9 mm.

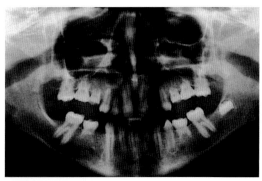

Fig. 32.1 Severe hypodontia. Source: Millett and Welbury 2000.

- Poor prognosis b|b . As spaces concern Ellen, consider extraction of b|b and replacement with an upper partial denture with prosthetic 2|2 .
- In adulthood the option of implants to replace the missing maxillary and mandibular teeth.

Case 2
Summary

Cameron was 3 when his mother brought him to the surgery because she was concerned that two of his teeth were joined together (**Fig. 32.2**). What is the cause and how may it be treated?

Medical and dental history

Cameron is an active child with no medical problems. He has no caries.

What can you see in Figure 32.2?

The crowns of the upper first and second primary incisors are joined.

A number of different terms have been used to describe the process of the formation of double teeth either on the primary or permanent dentitions: fusion, gemination, dichotomy, synodontia, schizodontia and connation. The mode of development given in older textbooks for the different names are unclear and unproven. The neutral term 'double teeth' is not contentious and describes accurately what the tooth looks like clinically.

How prevalent do you think double teeth are?

0.5–1.6% in primary dentition.

0.1–0.2% in permanent teeth.

No clear Mendelian trait established.

The clinical manifestation of the anomaly may vary considerably from a minor notch in the incisal edge of an abnormally wide incisor crown to the appearance of two separate crowns. There may be hard tissue continuity between either the crowns or the roots of the two elements or between both. Similarly there may be one unified pulp chamber and radicular pulp or separate ones.

In the primary dentition double teeth more commonly occur in the labial segments of the arches and most frequently in the mandible. Double permanent teeth can occur anywhere in the arch but are probably more frequent when involving incisors.

What are the most important clinical aspects of a double tooth in the primary dentition?

Caries may occur in the 'join' between the two coronal elements if it is not easily accessible to a toothbrush.

The presence of a numerical abnormality of the permanent dentition.

Counting a double tooth as one unit in the primary dentition, with relation to the total number of teeth present, may be helpful in predicting the type of numerical

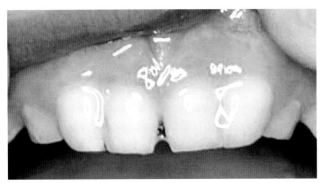

Fig. 32.2 Double incisor teeth.

abnormality of the permanent dentition. Hypodontia is usually followed by missing permanent teeth. A normal number of teeth in the primary dentition is often associated with permanent supernumeraries. The overall frequency of permanent numerical abnormalities following primary double teeth is between 30% and 50% in Caucasians and 75% in the Japanese population.

Radiography is therefore important at an appropriate time, so the parent can be advised of future treatment and prognosis and a treatment plan formulated. Extraction of double primary teeth may be necessary if physiological root resorption is significantly retarded. Surgical removal of supernumerary teeth may be required in order to facilitate eruption of normal units.

Key point

Double primary teeth may:
- Be associated with numerical abnormalities of the permanent dentition.
- Be a caries risk.
- Not undergo normal physiological resorption.

What are the important factors that will dictate whether you retain or extract double permanent teeth?

Space in the arch.
Aesthetics.
Morphology of pulp chambers and roots.
If the coronal parts of the double teeth are joined but the roots are separate, then it may be feasible to divide the crown and extract one portion of the crown and its root, thereby retaining the other portion of the crown with its root. The retained portion will require root canal treatment and subsequent coronal restoration.

What other types of crown abnormality do you know?

Accessory cusps.
Invaginations.
Evaginations.

Additional primary cusps are seen on the mesiobuccal aspect of maxillary first molars and the mesiopalatal aspect of maxillary second molars.

The commonest additional cusp in permanent teeth is often on the lingual cingulum, more commonly in the maxilla than the mandible. The name 'talon cusp' is often given to the additional cusp (**Fig. 32.3**). The cusp is composed of enamel, dentine and a horn of pulp tissue. Talons in maxillary anterior teeth like those in Figure 33.6 can cause a number of problems:

Appearance.
Occlusal interference.
Caries in the deep grooves between the cusp and the tooth.

The commonest accessory cusp in the permanent dentition is the mesiopalatal sited tubercle of Carabelli on the maxillary first molar (10–60%).

What are the treatment options for a talon cusp on a maxillary tooth?

Selective grinding of cusp to encourage obliteration of the pulp horn by secondary dentine.
Aseptic removal of the cusp under rubber dam followed by a limited pulpotomy procedure (immature or mature root).
Aseptic removal of cusp and one-stage endodontic treatment (mature root).

Failure of a pulpotomy technique in an immature tooth will result in the need for induced apical closure with non-setting calcium hydroxide. Many clinicians favour waiting until full root formation has occurred prior to removal of the cusp. Invaginations or invagination of the enamel epithelium into the dental papilla of the underlying tooth germ has been described as 'dens in dente', 'gestant composite odontome' and 'dilated composite odontome'. The correct descriptive term is 'dens invaginatus' or 'invaginated tooth'. The anomaly may vary clinically from a deep cingulum pit in a tooth of normal form (**Fig. 32.4**) to a tooth with grossly distorted crown and root. Invaginated teeth are relatively common, occurring in 1–5% of permanent teeth. Primary invaginations are rare.

The main problem with invaginations is infection. The enamel lining of the invagination is either incomplete or very thin and easily breached, resulting in dentinal caries that quickly progresses to involve the pulp causing a rapidly spreading infection presenting with acute facial cellulitis or acute dentoalveolar abscess. Rarely a large invaginated tooth may cause impaction and non-eruption of an adjacent tooth.

There is an association between invaginated teeth and supernumerary teeth. A full radiographic examination is justified if an invaginated tooth is identified.

Invaginations in crowns of normal morphology should be sealed prophylactically as soon as possible after

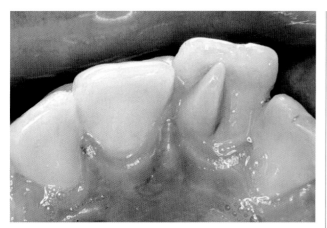

Fig. 32.3 Talon cusp.

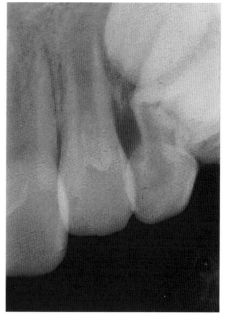

Fig. 32.4 Dens in dente of lateral incisor.

eruption. If these 'high' invaginations do become pulpally involved then root treatment is possible, because the invaginated portion is accessible and can be removed with a crown bur allowing access to the normal root canal. All other invaginations usually require extraction.

'Evaginated teeth' or 'dens evaginatus' or 'tuberculated teeth' occurs commonly as a conical tubercular projection arising from the occlusal surface of the central fissure or the lingual plane of the buccal cusp. Premolar teeth are the commonest teeth affected, with permanent molars and canines less common. The condition is mainly seen in people of Mongolian stock (1–4%), although rarely it is seen in Caucasians.

Evaginations consist of enamel, dentine and a pulpal extension. Evagination should be suspected if a premolar without caries develops a periapical lesion shortly after eruption.

Treatment is the same as 'talon cusp'.

What abnormalities of root form do you know?

Taurodontism.
Accessory roots.
Pyramidal roots.

Taurodontism (bull-like teeth) applies to multirooted teeth in which the body of the tooth is enlarged coronoapically at the expense of the roots. Radiographs show apparent enlargement of the coronal pulp chamber, usually extending below the level of the alveolar crest before root division. The normal constriction at the level of the amelocemental junction is frequently absent in affected teeth. The condition is uncommon in primary teeth but may occur in permanent molars in 6% of the population.

What conditions may taurodontism be associated with?

Amelogenesis imperfecta.
Trichodento-osseous syndrome.
Ectodermal dysplasia with hypodontia.
Ellis–van Creveld syndrome.
Achondroplasia.
Klinefelter's syndrome.

Accessory roots can occur in almost any tooth. Rarely they may be due to early trauma in a forming root. The majority are likely to be due to genetic factors that remain to be specified.

Pyramidal roots describe the reduction in root number in multirooted teeth. Any molar tooth may be affected.

Recommended reading

Cameron A, Widmer R (eds) 2003 Dental anomalies. In: Handbook of pediatric dentistry, 2nd edn. Mosby-Wolfe, St Louis, pp 184–192.

Millett D, Welbury R 2000 Orthodontics and paediatric dentistry. A colour guide. Churchill Livingstone, Edinburgh.

Winter GB 2001 Anomalies of tooth formation and eruption. In: Welbury RR (ed) Paediatric dentistry, 2nd edn. Oxford University Press, Oxford, pp 271–298.

For revision see Mind Map 32, page 178

33

Amelogenesis imperfecta

Summary

Mark is 10. He and his parents are concerned because his teeth seem rough. They also stain easily. What is the cause of these problems? What treatment is possible?

What can you see in Figure 33.1?
History

Mark's mother says that she noticed when the teeth first erupted that they were rough. They pick up stain and are difficult to clean. What key questions do you need to ask?

Was there any systemic illness from birth to early childhood?

No.

Were the primary teeth similarly affected?

There was a slight roughening of the primary teeth, although nothing as bad as the permanent teeth.

Is anyone else in the family similarly affected?

Mark's father and his cousin (father's brother's son) have similar roughness of their teeth.

After having obtained this history it is most likely that Mark has an inherited enamel defect involving enamel—amelogenesis imperfecta. However, defective enamel formation may be caused by genetic or environmental factors. The defective enamel will exhibit either hypoplasia, due to deficient matrix production, or hypominerali-zation, from imperfect mineralization of the matrix proteins. In hypoplasia the enamel may be thin, grooved or pitted, whereas in hypomineralization it may appear mottled but of normal thickness. The complete range of the causes of developmental abnormalities of enamel are shown in **Box 33.1**

Enamel defects of genetic origin may occur either as a phenomenon primarily involving the enamel, with possible secondary effects in other dental tissues and craniofacial structures, or as a component of a more complex syndrome in which defective enamel is only one of a number of more generalized abnormalities.

● Medical history

Mark has no medical problems. He is doing very well at school and is a keen basketball player.

Examination

Intraoral examination revealed that all the surfaces of all the erupted permanent teeth are affected by a roughness or 'pitting' (Fig. 33.1). The second primary molar teeth that were still present were also affected by a similar roughness that, although not as evident on visual examination, was obvious on tactile examination with a probe. There was no tooth wear.

Why is this pattern of enamel hypoplasia unlikely to be caused by systemic (chronological) influences?

Primary teeth were affected.

All the enamel surface of the teeth is affected.

Amelogenesis imperfecta (AI) occurs as a result of single gene mutations that follow autosomal-dominant, autosomal-recessive or X-linked patterns of inheritance. The prevalence varies around the world with rates of 1 in 718 in northern Sweden and 1 in 14 000 in Michigan USA. A global quoted figure is often 1 in 10 000.

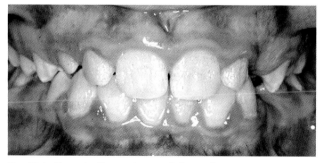

Fig. 33.1 Hypoplastic amelogenesis imperfecta.

> **Box 33.1** Developmental abnormalities of enamel
>
> **General factors**
> 1. Genetic
>   (a) primarily involving enamel—amelogenesis imperfecta
>   (b) associated with generalized defects
> 2. Systemic (chronological)
>   (a) nutritional deficiencies
>   (b) metabolic or biochemical disorder
>   (c) toxic substances
>   (d) infectious illnesses: prenatal; perinatal; neonatal; infancy; early childhood
> 3. Idiopathic
>
> **Local factors**
> 1. Trauma
> 2. Infection

What are the main types of AI?

- Hypoplastic.
- Hypomineralized:
  hypocalcified
  hypomature.
- 'Mixed'.

Currently there are about 14 different types of AI on the basis of genetic pattern, clinical and radiological features, and histological changes. These are shown in **Table 33.1**.

Genetic enamel defects can be associated with generalized disorders in a number of uncommon or rare genetically determined diseases and clinical syndromes. These diseases and complex syndromes include epidermolysis bullosa, tuberose sclerosis, pseudohypoparathyroidism, trichodento-osseous syndrome, oculodento-osseous dysplasia, vitamin D-dependent rickets, amelo-cerebrohypohidrotic syndrome, amelo-onychohypohidrotic syndrome and some types of mucopolysaccharidosis.

Mark probably has type 1B, autosomal-dominant, thin and rough hypoplasia. An example of a hypomature form of AI is shown in **Figure 33.2**.

Investigations

What investigations are necessary?

Dental panoramic tomogram. This will confirm the presence of all the permanent dentition. In addition it will diagnose any taurodontism. This is

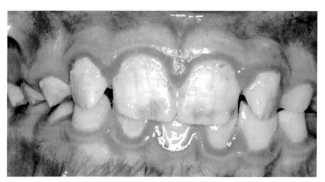

Fig. 33.2 Hypomature amelogenesis imperfecta.

most marked in type IV AI but can affect permanent molars, particularly in the maxilla in other types of AI more frequently than is the norm for the Caucasian population.

Family examination. If it is possible to examine Mark's father's and his cousin's teeth this will help to confirm your diagnosis.

Treatment

The treatment of both amelogenesis and dentinogenesis imperfecta requires early diagnosis in order to improve the long-term prognosis of teeth. Parents need to be educated as to the implications of the condition, and prevention (diet counselling, fluoride supplementation, oral hygiene instruction (OHI)) is a crucial element in the success of any restorative treatment.

There are four main clinical problems associated with inherited enamel and dentine defects:

Poor aesthetics.

Chipping and attrition of the enamel.

Exposure and attrition of the dentine causing sensitivity.

Poor oral hygiene, gingivitis and caries.

While it is impossible to draw up a definitive treatment plan for all cases, it is possible to define the principles of treatment planning for this group of patients. It is important to realize that not all children with amelogenesis imperfecta or dentinogenesis imperfecta are affected equally. Many will not have marked tooth wear or symptoms, and will not require advanced intervention. **Table 33.2** describes the principles of treatment in terms of the age of the child/adolescent and with regard to the three aspects of care: prevention, restoration and aesthetics.

Table 33.1 Types of amelogenesis imperfecta	
Type	**Description**
Type 1	*Hypoplasia*
1A	Autosomal-dominant, thin and smooth hypoplasia with eruption defect
1B	Autosomal-dominant, thin and rough hypoplasia
1C	Autosomal-dominant, randomly pitted hypoplasia
1D	Autosomal-dominant, localized hypoplasia
1E	Autosomal-recessive, localized hypoplasia
1F	X-linked hypoplasia
1G	Autosomal-recessive, thin and rough hypoplasia (agenesis)
Type II	*Hypocalcification*
IIA	Autosomal-dominant, hypocalcification
IIB	Autosomal-recessive, hypocalcification
Type III	*Hypomaturation*
IIIA	X-linked hypomaturation
IIIB	Autosomal-recessive, pigmented hypomaturation
IIIC	Autosomal-dominant, snow-capped teeth
Type IV	*Hypomaturation–hypoplasia with taurodontism*
IVA	Autosomal-dominant, hypomaturation with pitted hypoplasia and taurodontism
IVB	Autosomal-dominant, hypomaturation with thin hypoplasia and taurodontism

Key point

Main treatment aims for dental anomalies:
- To alleviate symptoms.
- To maintain/restore occlusal height.
- To improve aesthetics.

Mark's major concern was the staining and roughness of his front teeth. Fortunately there was no wear of his posterior teeth and his problem, therefore, was solely a cosmetic one. The pitting or hypoplasia on the upper and lower incisors can be masked by a thin directly applied composite veneer. This should be extended to include the canines and first premolars when the arches are complete. On occasions, if the smile is a very 'wide' one, it may be necessary to include second premolars. Composite veneers can be replaced by porcelain veneers at age 18 when the gingival contour has achieved adult levels.

If the amelogenesis had been of the hypomineralized variety with more destruction of enamel, it may have been necessary to consider full porcelain crowns for aesthetics in the anterior teeth and either stainless steel crowns or adhesive castings on posterior teeth. The latter may need to be replaced in adolescence/early adulthood by a porcelain bonded full crown (Table 34.2).

Table 33.2 Treatment modalities for amelogenesis imperfecta

	Restoration	Aesthetics
Primary dentition 0–5 years	Adhesive restorations Stainless steel crowns (SSCs) especially on e's	Minimal intervention Compomer/ composite veneers
Mixed dentition 6–16 years	Adhesive restorations/ SSCs on primary molars SSCs/adhesive castings on permanent molars	Composite veneers
Permanent dentition 16+ years	Adhesive castings on premolars Full mouth rehabilitation ± crown lengthening	Porcelain veneers Full crowns

Recommended reading

Cameron A, Widmer R (eds) 2003 Dental anomalies. In: Handbook of paediatric dentistry. 2nd edn. Mosby-Wolfe, St Louis, pp 213–218.
Winter GB 2001 Anomalies of tooth formation and eruption. In: Welbury RR (ed) Paediatric dentistry, 2nd edn. Oxford University Press, Oxford, pp 271–298.

For revision see Mind Map 33, page 179

34

Dentinogenesis imperfecta

Summary

Siobhan is 9. She and her parents are concerned because her permanent teeth are darker than normal and she is getting teased at school. What is the cause of the discoloration? How would you treat it?

History

Siobhan's mother says she noticed that when the permanent teeth erupted they looked darker. Siobhan is very unhappy at school and refuses to smile for any photographs. When she talks she has the habit of covering her mouth with a hand so it is impossible to see her teeth. What can you see in **Figure 34.1a**? What key questions do you need to ask?

Was there any systemic illness from birth until early childhood?

No. Siobhan had no illness.

Were the primary teeth similarly affected?

The primary teeth erupted normally but very quickly chipped away becoming worn to gum level

Is anyone else in the family similarly affected?

Siobhan's brother and her father have a problem with their teeth. Siobhan's brother is 14 and he has needed crowns on his back teeth and veneers on his front teeth. Siobhan's father needed a lot of treatment when he was younger and has had some teeth crowned. Many of his posterior teeth, however, were extracted.

Even before you have examined the mouth your history suggests that Siobhan has an inherited defect. Figure 34.1a confirms your suspicion that this is dentinogenesis imperfecta (DI).

Why is this DI and not amelogenesis imperfecta (AI)?

The teeth are translucent.

The enamel is poorly adherent to the underlying dentine and easily chips and wears. The remaining primary canines and molars in **Figures 35.1a** and **b** are worn to gingival level and have a translucent opalescent appearance.

What investigations do you need to do to confirm your suspicions?

Dental panoramic tomogram. If this is DI it will probably show the following:

Bulbous crowns with pronounced cervical constriction.

Shortened roots.

Progressive pulp chamber and canal obliteration (**Fig. 34.2** (different case)).

Spontaneous periapical abscess formation.

Family examination of affected members.

Dentine defects like those of enamel may be subdivided by cause into two main groups based on whether they are of genetic or environmental origin.

Dentine anomalies that are genetically determined may appear to be limited to the dentition or form part of a more complex generalized disorder (**Box 34.1**).

The most well documented hereditary dentine defects are DI type II (hereditary opalescent dentine), which only

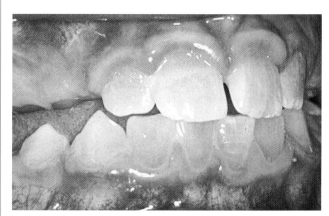

Fig. 34.1 a

Fig. 34.1 b

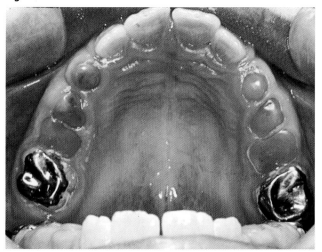

Fig. 34.1 (a,b) Dentinogenesis imperfecta.

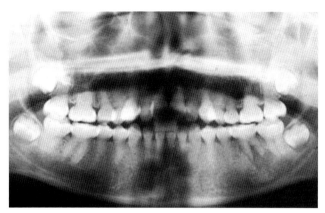

Fig. 34.2 Obliteration of root canals and pulp chambers in dentinogenesis imperfecta.

affects teeth, and DI type I, in which abnormalities of teeth are associated with osteogenesis imperfecta.

● DI type II

Both dentitions are usually affected. The severity of the defect varies considerably between families and within families. Primary teeth tend to be more severely affected than permanent teeth and the later forming permanent teeth may be the least affected. Enamel tends to chip away from the underlying amelodentinal junction (ADJ) exposing the abnormally soft dentine that undergoes rapid wear. This is most marked in the primary dentition where, within 2 years, the crowns may be worn to the gingival margin and appear as amber-coloured remnants (Fig. 34.1b), which may be frequently infected and abscessed. In the permanent dentition following eruption the enamel may look reasonably normal, but histological studies have shown hypomineralized areas in approximately one-third of cases. Radiographic signs are mentioned above. Histologically the ADJ may appear flattened, and while the subadjacent peripheral dentine may approach normality, the remainder is grossly disordered with an amorphous matrix containing areas of interglobular calcification, abnormally shaped and sized tubules, and cellular inclusions.

Box 34.1 Hereditary dentine defects

1. Limited to the dentine:
   (a) dentinogenesis imperfecta type II (hereditary opalescent dentine)
   (b) dentine dysplasia type I (radicular dentine dysplasia)
   (c) dentine dysplasia type II (coronal dentine dysplasia)
   (d) fibrous dysplasia of dentine
2. Associated with generalized disorder:
   (a) osteogenesis imperfecta (dentinogenesis imperfecta type I)
   (b) Ehlers–Danlos syndrome
   (c) brachioskeletogenital syndrome
   (d) vitamin D-resistant rickets
   (e) vitamin D-dependent rickets
   (f) hypophosphatasia

Is DI more prevalent than AI?

Possibly. Figures of 1 in 8000 have been estimated (AI 1 : 10 000).

Has DI got as many inheritance patterns as AI?

No. Invariably it is autosomal-dominant with marked expressivity and good penetrance. Two clinical variants of the condition have been described:

Shell teeth. This is rare and seen in the primary dentition. The pulp remains large and the thin enamel and dentine rapidly fragments to cause pulpal infection.

DI type III (brandy wine type). This was first described in Maryland USA and has been traced back to East Anglia in England. It was apparently taken to the USA by one of the sailors who accompanied the Pilgrim Fathers to Maryland. More recently type III defect has been linked to the same locus on chromosome 4q21 as DI type II.

● DI type I associated with osteogenesis imperfecta

Osteogenesis imperfecta is a group of connective tissue disorders involving inherited abnormalities of type I collagen. Increased bone fragility is only one aspect of the condition which may include lax joints, blue sclerae, opalescent teeth, hearing loss and a variable degree of bone deformity. The inheritance pattern is either autosomal recessive or dominant. The recessive form is often lethal around birth.

Opalescent teeth are only rarely seen in surviving recessive types. They are commonly a feature of the dominant variety with accompanying bone fragility, bone deformity and blue sclerae.

The primary teeth in DI type I resemble exactly those in DI type II. However, in the permanent dentition the defect is extremely variable. In many cases the upper anterior teeth may have a normal colour and appearance whereas the lower incisors and canines are opalescent, discoloured bluish-brown and wear at the incisal edges. In most cases the enamel does not chip away from underlying dentine as readily as in type II.

Radiographic appearances are as already described with the exception that upper teeth may retain their pulp spaces long after those in the lower jaw. Histological appearances are indistinguishable from type II.

Environmentally determined dentine defects do exist but are less well documented than corresponding anomalies of enamel. Trauma; nutritional deficiencies of minerals, proteins and vitamins; drugs—tetracycline; chemotherapeutic agents—cyclophosphamide, will likely produce increased interglobular dentine, predentine and osteoid.

Key point

Dentinogenesis imperfecta:
- Occurs in 1 in 8000 of the population.
- May be associated with osteogenesis imperfecta.

Treatment

The main clinical problems associated with AI and DI, and the key points of treatment objectives are covered in Chapter 33.

The principles of treatment for DI are the same as those for AI with the exception that in the permanent dentition from age 16 crown-lengthening procedures are more common in DI and the provision of overdentures and full dentures is not uncommon. The role of implants in these patients has yet to be defined.

Siobhan's major concern was of the colour of her permanent incisors. There was some wear of first permanent molars. The first permanent molars were treated with adhesive castings with micromechanical retention to luting cement (Fig. 34.1b). The upper and lower incisors were veneered with composite resin. This can be extended to include the canines and premolars when the arches are complete. The composite veneers can be replaced by porcelain veneers around the age of 18 years.

Young children with DI often pose the greatest problems. The teeth undergo such excessive wear that they become worn down to gingival level and are unrestorable. Teeth affected by DI are also prone to spontaneous abscesses due to the progressive obliteration of the pulp chambers. In these cases pulp therapy is unsuccessful and extraction of the affected teeth is necessary.

Early consultation with an orthodontist is advisable in inherited abnormalities of enamel and dentine in order to keep the orthodontic requirements simple. Treatment for these patients is possible and in many cases proceeds without problems. The use of removable appliances, where appropriate, and orthodontic bands rather than brackets will minimize the risk of damage to the abnormal enamel. The problem is twofold: there may be frequent bond failure during active treatment or the enamel may be further damaged during debonding. Some orthodontists prefer to use bands even for anterior teeth, while others will use glass ionomer cement as the bonding agent in preference to more conventional resin-based agents. In other instances, cosmetic restorative techniques (veneers and crowns) may be more appropriate than orthodontic treatment.

Recommended reading

Cameron A, Widmer R (eds) 2003 Dental anomalies. In: Handbook of paediatric dentistry, 2nd edn. Mosby-Wolfe, St Louis, pp 218–223.

Winter GB 2001 Anomalies of tooth formation and eruption. In: Welbury RR(ed) Paediatric dentistry, 2nd edn. Oxford University Press, Oxford, pp 271–298.

For revision see Mind Map 34, page 180

35

Gingival bleeding and enlargement

Summary

Kayleigh is 15. She is concerned that her upper gums look abnormal and they bleed whenever she brushes them (**Fig. 35.1**).

History

Kayleigh has noticed bleeding when she has been brushing for the last year. She is frightened of brushing because of the bleeding and feels that the bleeding is getting worse. She is also very socially conscious of her gums because they look very red and are 'bigger' than normal.

Medical history

Kayleigh is an insulin-dependent diabetic. She takes her insulin by subcutaneous injection at 07.30 and 17.30 hours. She has a regulated gram intake of carbohydrate at 07.30, 11.00, 13.00, 15.00, 17.30 and 21.00. Apart from this she is an active girl who plays basketball and hockey at school and has learnt to increase her carbohydrate intake appropriately to cover her sporting activities. Her mum reports that Kayleigh has had the occasional 'rebellion' against her condition and at these times diabetic control has been poor, but generally her control is now good with a stable regime. She is seen

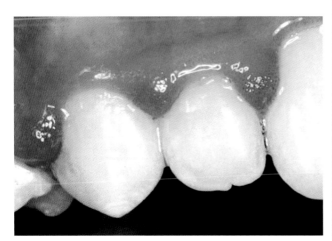

Fig. 35.1 Chronic gingivitis.

every 2 months by her doctor and monitors her blood glucose and urinary glucose at home herself.

Dental history

Kayleigh and her family are regular dental attenders and have just moved to the area with her father's job. This is the first time you have seen her.

Examination

Extraoral examination is normal with no signs of infection. Intraorally there is widespread marginal gingivitis, which is particularly bad in the upper right quadrant anteriorly (Fig. 35.1). Clinical and radiographic examination of the teeth reveal a low caries rate with only the need to replace a cracked and deficient restoration in a lower first permanent molar that has recurrent caries.

What factors are contributing to the chronic marginal gingivitis?

Poor oral hygiene.
Hormonal changes of puberty.
Poorly controlled diabetes mellitus.

> ### Key point
>
> Gingival bleeding can be as a result of:
> - Local causes.
> - Systemic causes.

The commonest local and systemic causes of gingival bleeding in childhood/adolescence are shown in **Box 35.1**.

Box 35.1 Commonest causes of gingival bleeding in childhood and adolescence

Local causes
- Eruption gingivitis
- Acute/chronic gingivitis
- Chronic periodontitis
- Foreign body entrapment
- Acute necrotizing ulcerative gingivitis
- Haemangioma
- Reactive hyperplasias such as pyogenic granuloma
- Factitial injury

Systemic causes:
- Hormonal changes such as pregnancy or puberty
- Diabetes mellitus—poor control
- Anaemia
- Leukaemia
- Any platelet disorder
- Clotting defects
- Drugs (e.g. anticoagulants)
- Scurvy
- HIV-associated periodontal disease

What do you think may have precipitated the initial gingivitis?

This is likely to have coincided with one of the periods where diabetic control was poor. Further questioning revealed that about a year ago Kayleigh was struggling to come to terms with her insulin-dependent diabetes. She refused to take her insulin regularly and ended up by being admitted to hospital in coma with ketoacidosis. Her blood sugar at that time was very high and her breath smelt of 'pear drops' due to ketone bodies. This was a hyperglycaemic coma. She was resuscitated with intravenous fluids as she was severely dehydrated, prior to restabilization on an insulin regime.

What is the other cause of diabetic coma and what are its signs?

Hypoglycaemic coma due to inadequate carbohydrate (missed meal), exercise or excess insulin. The onset is quicker than the hyperglycaemic coma. The signs of hypoglycaemic coma are very similar to having 'a drink too many', and can be summarized into those caused by adrenaline release and cerebral hypoglycaemia:

- Adrenaline release:
  - sweaty warm skin
  - rapid bounding pulse
  - dilated (reacting pupils)
  - anxiety, tremor
  - tingling around mouth.
- Cerebral hypoglycaemia:
  - confusion, disorientation
  - headache
  - dysarthria
  - unconsciousness
  - focal neurological signs, e.g. fits.

If the subject in a hypoglycaemic episode is conscious they should be given sugar orally—25 g glucose. If comatosed they require 20 mg of 20% dextrose IV followed by 25 g orally on arousal. Alternatively if IV access is difficult, 1 mg IM of glucagon. In practical terms 10 g glucose approximates to:

- 2 tsp sugar
- 3 lumps sugar
- 3 Dextrosol tablets
- 60 ml Lucozade
- 15 ml Ribena (full sugar type)
- 90 ml cola (not diet variety)
- one-third pint milk.

Treatment

Kayleigh's gingivitis probably started as a result of poor diabetic control and unfortunately has been compounded by poor oral hygiene and the hormonal changes of puberty.

Why is the gingivitis worst in the anterior part of the upper right quadrant?

She is right-handed and this is often the case when a right-handed person changes their brushing action from the left hand side of the mouth to the right hand side. The opposite would be true for the left-hander.

What other generalized causes of gingival enlargement do you know?

There are a number of causes that can be classified into congenital and acquired (**Box 35.2**).

Why is it important to eradicate Kayleigh's gingivitis?

Poor oral hygiene in combination with diabetes can result in rapid periodontal destruction and attachment loss. An example of this in another subject with diabetes is shown in **Figure 35.2**. There is some evidence that significant periodontitis can upset glycaemic control.

Box 35.2 Systemic causes of gingival enlargement

Congenital
- Hereditary gingival fibromatosis
- Mucopolysaccharidoses
- Infantile systemic hyalinosis

Acquired
- Puberty/pregnancy gingivitis
- Plasma cell gingivitis
- Infections—HSV
- Haematological: acute myeloid leukaemia, preleukaemic leukaemia, aplastic anaemia, vitamin C deficiency (scurvy)
- Drugs: phenytoin, cyclosporin, calcium channel blockers, vigabatrin
- Deposits: mucocutaneous amyloidosis
- Chronic granulomatous disorders: sarcoidosis, Crohn's disease, orofacial granulomatosis

---

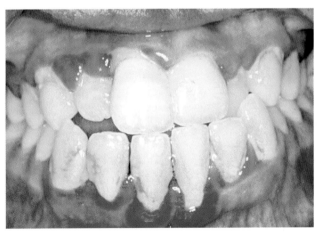

Fig. 35.2 Gingival and periodontal disease.

Kayleigh needs reassurance that the bleeding will reduce and stop when her oral hygiene improves. She needs to appreciate the importance of good oral hygiene and the problems that will occur if oral hygiene is poor.

Why is it important not to leave caries in a diabetic?

Infection of any origin can result in an increased need for insulin. Without an insulin increase there will be a rise in blood sugar resulting in ketosis. Therefore, all infections in a diabetic, including those in the orofacial region, should be treated vigorously with antibiotics. Caries should be treated early to prevent infection.

Key point

In diabetes:
- Poor oral hygiene will accelerate attachment loss.
- Infection can interfere with diabetic control.

Why is the timing of the appointment to restore Kayleigh's first permanent molar important?

So you do not interfere with her carbohydrate intake and precipitate hypoglycaemia. It is probably best to give her an appointment either first thing in the morning, or directly after lunch. For any prolonged surgical procedure in a diabetic or any treatment that requires general anaesthesia (GA), then a referral to hospital is required. GA will require admission preoperatively to stabilize insulin and glucose requirements via a drip in order that hypoglycaemic coma does not occur with preoperative GA starvation.

What dietary advice should you give to diabetic patients?

Do not change your required carbohydrate intakes as these are critical to diabetic control.

Tailor the dental advice to the specific needs of the patient, i.e. take your toothbrush to school if possible. Try to clean your teeth after snacks and at lunchtime. Try to take snacks that provide the necessary sugar but don't remain stuck to the teeth. Use sugar-free gum if it is not possible to brush the teeth during the day.

What other oral manifestations can occur in diabetes?

Dry mouth.
Swelling of salivary glands (sialosis).
Glossitis.
Burning of tongue.
Oral candidosis if control is poor.

These manifestations are more commonly seen in adults.

Recommended reading

Firatli E, Yilmaz O, Onan U 1996 The relationship between clinical attachment loss and the duration of insulin dependent diabetes mellitus (IDDM) in children and adolescents. J Clin Periodontol 23:362–366.

Karjalainen KM, Knuuttila MLE, Kaar M-L 1997 Relationship between caries and level of metabolic balance in children and adolescents with insulin-dependent diabetes mellitus. Caries Res 31:13–18.

Position paper 1996 Diabetes and periodontal diseases. J Periodontol 67:166–176.

For revision see Mind Map 35, page 181

36
Oral ulceration

Summary

Alan is 8. He has been brought to the surgery by his mother because his mouth is so painful he cannot eat (**Fig. 36.1**). What could cause this problem? How would you treat it?

History

Alan has not been well for a couple of weeks. He had a 'virus' that resulted in his being put to bed and missing school. Just as he was improving from this his mouth became very sore. He has been unable to eat solid food for 3 days and has been on liquids only. He feels hot and lethargic. His gums bleed when he tries to brush them.

Medical history

Alan is generally a healthy boy. He has had a couple of courses of antibiotics for ear infections but has had no real illnesses. He has never been in hospital and is not on any tablets or medicines from his doctor.

Describe the appearance of the upper and lower gingivae in Figure 36.1.

There is erythematous gingival enlargement with small ulcerations of the gingival margin.

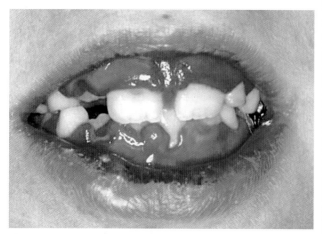

Fig. 36.1 Gingival enlargement and ulceration.

What is the diagnosis?

Primary herpetic gingivostomatitis.

There are two types of herpes simplex virus: herpes simplex type 1 (HSV-1) and herpes simplex type 2 (HSV-2). Classically HSV-1 causes oral disease and HSV-2 genital disease. The viruses, however, are very similar and both can cause both oral and genital disease, although there are differences in recurrence rates. Primary exposure to HSV in the mouth causes acute primary herpetic gingivostomatitis (Fig. 36.1). The virus causes a viraemia, fever, malaise and lymphadenopathy. All the surfaces of the mouth including the hard palate and attached gingiva can be involved, initially with a vesicular rash that ulcerates and becomes superinfected. The illness lasts for 10–14 days before resolving spontaneously. Diagnosis is usually made on clinical grounds but can be confirmed by a threefold rise in the convalescent antibody titre over that seen in the acute phase or by direct immuno-fluorescence of vesicular fluid using specific antisera.

> ### Key point
>
> Systemic signs in HSV:
> - Fever.
> - Malaise.
> - Lymphadenopathy.

The primary infection may be mild and subclinical in the majority of young children who are exposed to it, though the condition may be severe and debilitating, and in an immunocompromised individual may lead to severe illness and sometimes herpetic hepatitis or encephalitis, which may be fatal in the absence of treatment.

Oral infection arises from direct contact with secretions from an individual who either has a primary or recurrent HSV infection. Direct inoculation of the fingers or skin with virally contaminated secretions or fluid can lead to local infection, e.g. herpetic whitlow of finger.

HSV is a neurogenic virus, and on recovery from the primary infection the virus may become latent within the trigeminal ganglion or basal ganglia of the brain and may subsequently be reactivated to cause a secondary infection. The secondary infection may cause a 'cold sore' on the lip or Bell's palsy.

Treatment

Alan responded well to rehydration and analgesia such as paracetamol, which is also antipyretic, and an antiseptic mouthwash such as chlorhexidine (corsodyl) or benzydamine hydrochloride (Difflam). Had Alan not been able to maintain hydration he would have had to be admitted for intravenous fluid therapy. There is no evidence that systemic acyclovir is of any benefit at the relatively late stage of the condition that he presented. If he had been seen within 72 hours of the onset of the infection then acyclovir could have been prescribed, if the clinical severity warranted it, at a dose of 200 mg five times daily for 5 days in over 2 years of age, and 100 mg five times daily for 2 days in the under 2 year olds. Although acyclovir can shorten the course of the primary infection, there is no evidence that it reduces the incidence of recurrent herpetic lesions.

What are the reasons given for the reactivation of HSV to produce a cold sore (herpes labialis) (Fig. 36.2)?

See **Table 36.1**.

How should herpes labialis be treated?

Apply acyclovir 5% cream to the lip lesion as soon as tingling or prickling of the prodromal phase is felt. This is usually 24 hours prior to vesculation and pain.

What other viral infection can occur in the mouths of paediatric patients?

● Varicella-zoster virus (VZV)

VZV is a neurogenic DNA virus that causes a primary infection in the form of chickenpox. Thereafter it remains dormant until reactivation as shingles.

● Epstein-Barr virus (EBV)

EBV is a herpes virus with a predilection for infecting B-lymphocytes. This infection causes the B-lymphocytes to become activated and produce their own antibody. A primary infection with EBV causes glandular fever or infectious mononucleosis.

● Cytomegalovirus

This is associated with a glandular fever-like illness in childhood. On occasion it is found in severe atypical oral ulceration in HIV.

● Herpes virus type 8

This has been demonstrated in Kaposi's sarcoma in HIV.

● Coxsackie viruses

These are RNA viruses and responsible for herpangina or hand, foot and mouth disease.

Herpangina is a Coxsackie A virus that causes a herpes-like oropharyngitis where the ulceration is

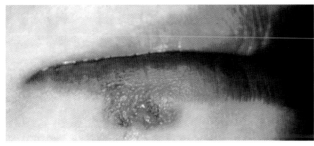

Fig. 36.2 Recurrent herpes 'cold sore'.

<table>
<tr><td>Box 36.1 Reactivation of HSV</td></tr>
<tr><td>

● Trauma
● Chemicals
● Heat
● Hormones
● Sunlight
● Emotion
● Immunosuppression
● Concurrent infection

</td></tr>
</table>

predominantly on the tonsil, soft palate and uvula. The mild illness is associated with fever and malaise but only persists for a few days.

Hand, foot and mouth disease is also Coxsackie A virus and occurs predominantly in children and throughout families. The condition is characterized by ulceration affecting gingiva, tongue, cheeks and palate. It is associated with vesicles and ulcers on the palms and soles. It may persist for 2 weeks.

● Human papilloma viruses

An increasing number of HPV types have been identified. Types 2 and 4, the common wart, occur in children usually due to autoinoculation by biting finger or hand warts. Condyloma acuminata or venereal warts can occur on the oral mucosa and are associated with HPV types 6, 11, 60.

There are a number of other causes of oral ulceration in children and adolescents that are not associated with infections. These are shown in **Table 36.2**.

What types of aphthae are there?

Minor.
Major.
Herpetiform.
Behçets.

Recurrent aphthae affect up to 20% of the population.

Minor aphthae are commonest and account for 85% of recurrent aphthae. Ulcers are less than 1 cm in diameter, usually only 2–3 mm. They occur singly or in crops of up to 10, last 3 days to 3 weeks and heal without scarring. Ulcers are round or oval with a yellowish-grey base and surrounded by an erythematous halo. They affect only non-keratinized mucosa.

Major aphthae are more severe and usually more than 1 cm in diameter with an irregular outline. They are usually single and often affect the fauces. They are often deeper and bleed, and may last for several weeks or months before healing with scarring. Again they tend to affect non-keratinized mucosa.

Herpetiform aphthae look similar to primary herpes. The ulcers are 1–2 mm in diameter and large numbers may occur simultaneously. They last from 2 days to 2

Box 36.2 Causes of oral ulceration

- Aphthae
- Gastrointestinal disease
- Haematological disease
- Infections
- Mucocutaneous disorders
- Radiotherapy
- Trauma
- Carcinoma

Box 36.3 Common aetiological factors in recurrent aphthae in children

Host factors
- Genetic
- Nutritional
- Systemic disease
- Immunity

Environmental factors
- Trauma
- Allergy
- Infection
- Stress

Key point

Aetiological factors in recurrent aphthae:
- Host related.
- Environment related.

---

shown in **Box 36.4**. Patients usually develop fresh ulceration within 12–24 hours of ingesting the suspect food. Foods may be identified more objectively by patch testing. Dietary avoidance is often attended by clinical improvement.

Treatment of recurrent aphthae can be grouped into preventive and symptomatic (**Box 36.5**).

Box 36.4 Common dietary allergens in recurrent aphthae

- Cheese
- Chocolate
- Nuts
- Tomatoes
- Citrus fruits
- Benzoates
- Cinnamon aldehyde

---

weeks before healing without scar formation. Again they affect only non-keratinized mucosa.

Behçet's syndrome describes the triad of oral and genital ulceration and anterior uveitis. Behçets is rare in the UK and USA.

What aetiological factors are important in recurrent aphthae?

See **Box 36.3**. Although only 20% of the population suffer from recurrent aphthae, there is a positive family history in 50% of fathers and 60% of mothers. There is, in addition, a weak HLA association with HLA types A2 and B_{12}.

Nutritional deficiencies of iron, folic acid and B_{12} occur singly or in combination. A lot of these are latent and have a normal peripheral blood picture. It is necessary to assay individual levels of ferritin, folic acid and vitamin B_{12} as well as do a full blood count (FBC).

What systemic diseases in children are commonly associated with aphthae?

Coeliac disease.

Crohn's disease.

Ulcerative colitis.

In older patients and less commonly in children, aphthae may also be associated with pernicious anaemia, HIV and malabsorption.

There is an increasing awareness of the role of dietary allergens in recurrent aphthae in children. Common dietary allergens implicated in recurrent aphthae are

---

Box 36.5 Therapy for recurrent aphthae

Preventive
- Haematinic replacement
- Dietary avoidance
- Tetracycline mouthwash
- Systemic corticosteroids
- Colchicine
- Thalidomide

Symptomatic
- Chlorhexidine mouthwash
- Benzydamine mouthwash
- Topical lidocaine (lignocaine) spray
- Topical lidocaine (lignocaine) ice lolly
- Topical 20% benzocaine to local ulcers
- Topical steroids:
    triamcinolone in dental paste
    beclomethasone inhaler spray
    betamethasone mouthwash

Recommended reading

Scully C, Porter SR 1989 Recurrent aphthous stomatitis: current concepts of etiology, pathogenesis and management. J Oral Pathol Med 18:21–27.

Scully C, Welbury R, Flaitz C, de Almeida OP 2002 A color atlas of orofacial health and disease in children and adolescents, 2nd edn. Martin Dunitz, London

Wray D, Rees SR, Gibson J, Forsyth A 2000 The role of allergy in oral mucosal diseases. Q J Med 93:507–511.

For revision see Mind Map 36, page 182

37
Mind Maps

How to use the Mind Maps

Within this chapter you will find Mind Maps relating to each of the previous chapters. For each topic:

1. Ensure that you have read through the topic in the main text twice.
2. Minutes after you have completed this, turn to the relevant Mind Map.
3. Use a highlighter or felt-tip pen to move around each Mind Map.
4. Link or isolate groups of words on the Mind Map with your highlighter or pen. Add cross-references to other maps and any additional points you wish to remember.
5. It may be useful to revise the Mind Map before going to bed as, in theory, the brain consolidates information during sleep.
6. Spend a few minutes the next day revising the Mind Map and test your recall of information.
7. At regular intervals revise the Mind Maps and make additions to them yourself following lectures and tutorials.

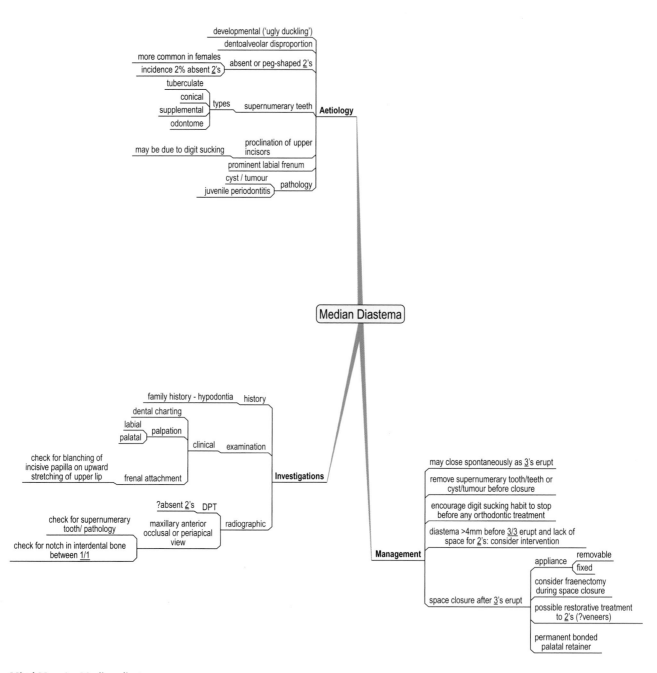

Mind Map 1a Median diastema

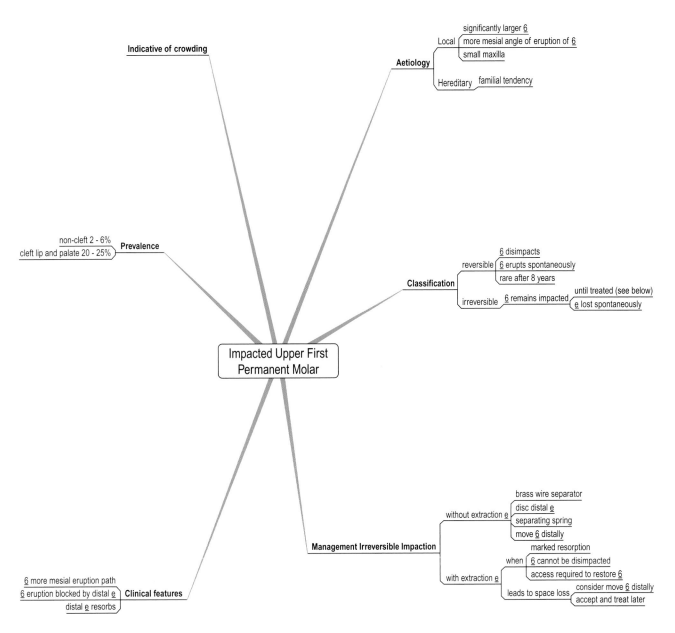

Mind Map 1b Impacted upper first permanent molar.

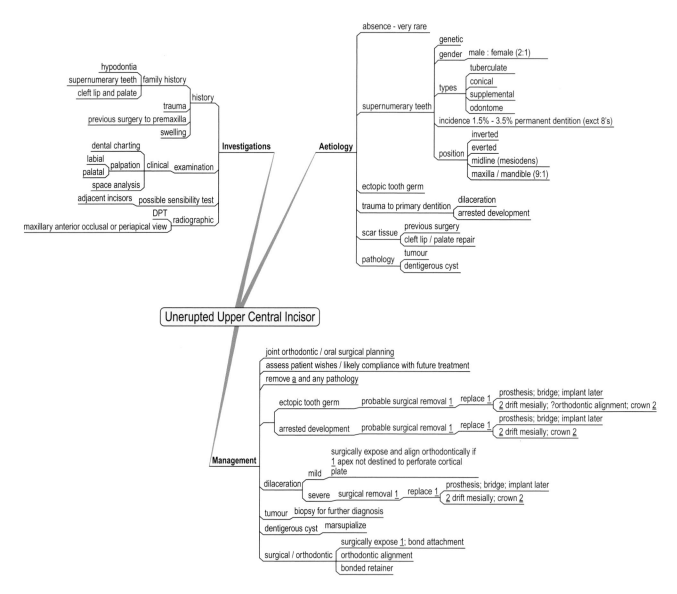

Mind Map 2 Unerupted upper central incisor.

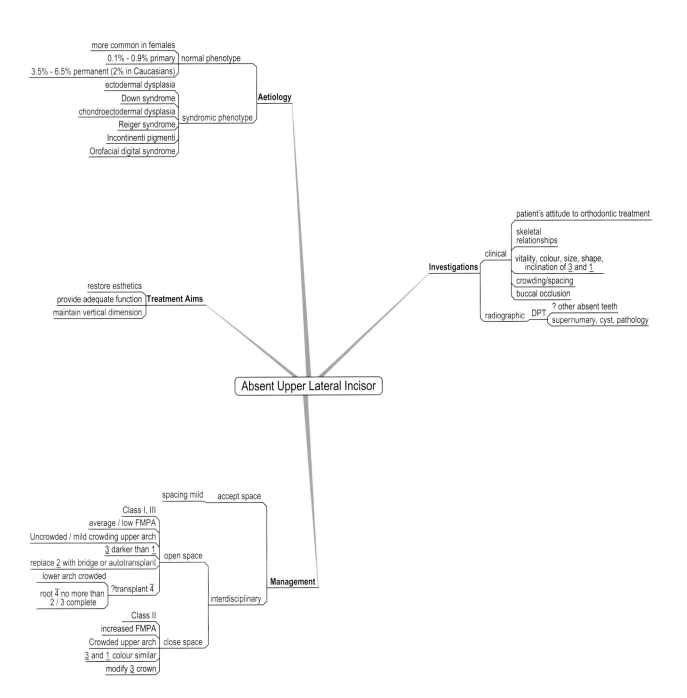

Mind Map 3 Absent upper lateral incisors.

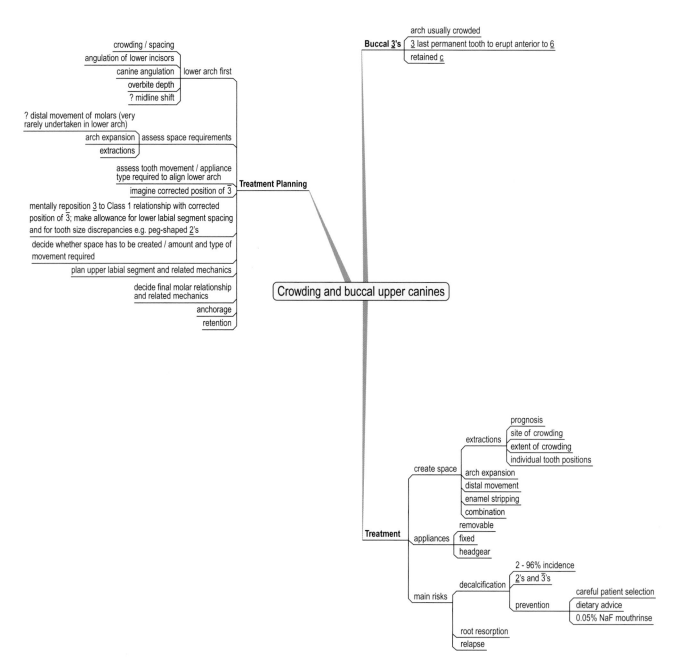

Mind Map 4 Crowding and buccal upper canines.

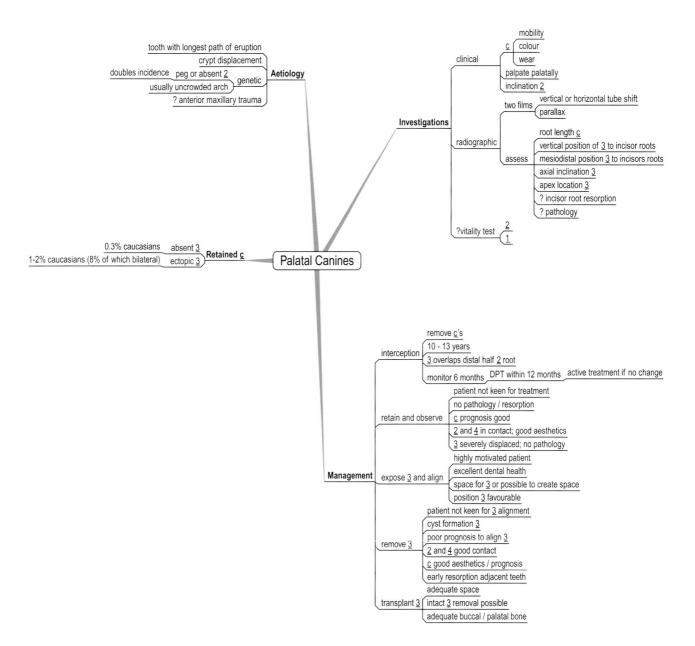

Mind Map 5 Palatal canines.

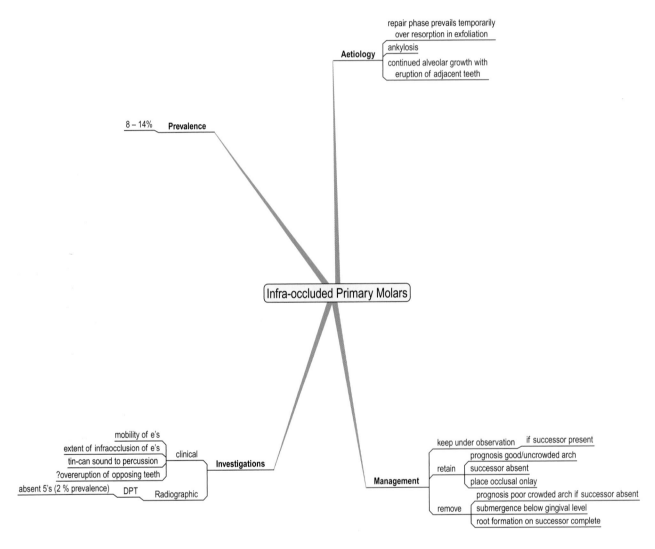

Mind Map 6 Infra-occluded primary molars.

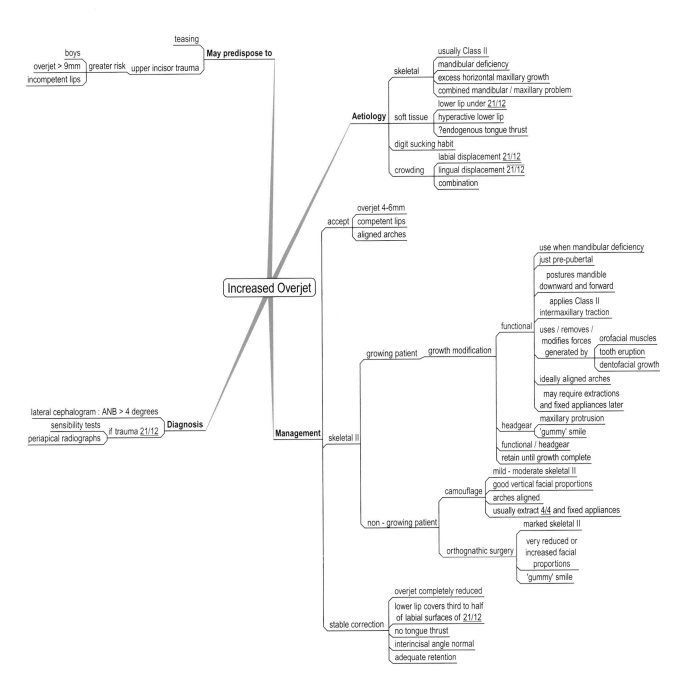

Increased Overjet

May predispose to — teasing
upper incisor trauma — greater risk — boys / overjet > 9mm / incompetent lips

Aetiology
- skeletal
  - usually Class II
  - mandibular deficiency
  - excess horizontal maxillary growth
  - combined mandibular / maxillary problem
- soft tissue
  - lower lip under 21/12
  - hyperactive lower lip
  - ?endogenous tongue thrust
- digit sucking habit
- crowding
  - labial displacement 21/12
  - lingual displacement 21/12
  - combination

Diagnosis
- lateral cephalogram : ANB > 4 degrees
- sensibility tests / periapical radiographs — if trauma 21/12

Management
- accept
  - overjet 4-6mm
  - competent lips
  - aligned arches
- skeletal II
  - growing patient — growth modification
    - functional
      - use when mandibular deficiency
      - just pre-pubertal
      - postures mandible downward and forward
      - applies Class II intermaxillary traction
      - uses / removes / modifies forces generated by — orofacial muscles / tooth eruption / dentofacial growth
      - ideally aligned arches
      - may require extractions and fixed appliances later
    - headgear
      - maxillary protrusion
      - 'gummy' smile
    - functional / headgear
    - retain until growth complete
  - non - growing patient
    - camouflage
      - mild - moderate skeletal II
      - good vertical facial proportions
      - arches aligned
      - usually extract 4/4 and fixed appliances
    - orthognathic surgery
      - marked skeletal II
      - very reduced or increased facial proportions
      - 'gummy' smile
- stable correction
  - overjet completely reduced
  - lower lip covers third to half of labial surfaces of 21/12
  - no tongue thrust
  - interincisal angle normal
  - adequate retention

Mind Map 7 Increased overjet.

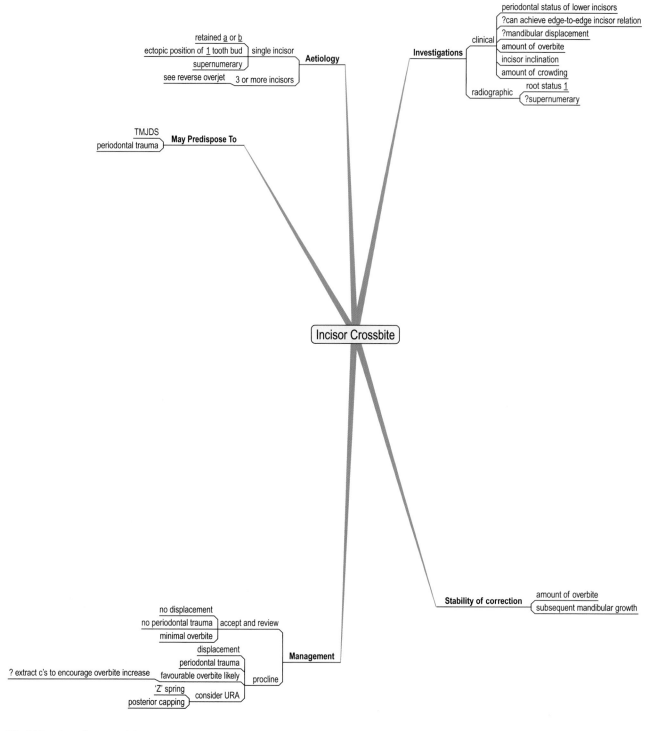

Mind Map 8 Incisor crossbite.

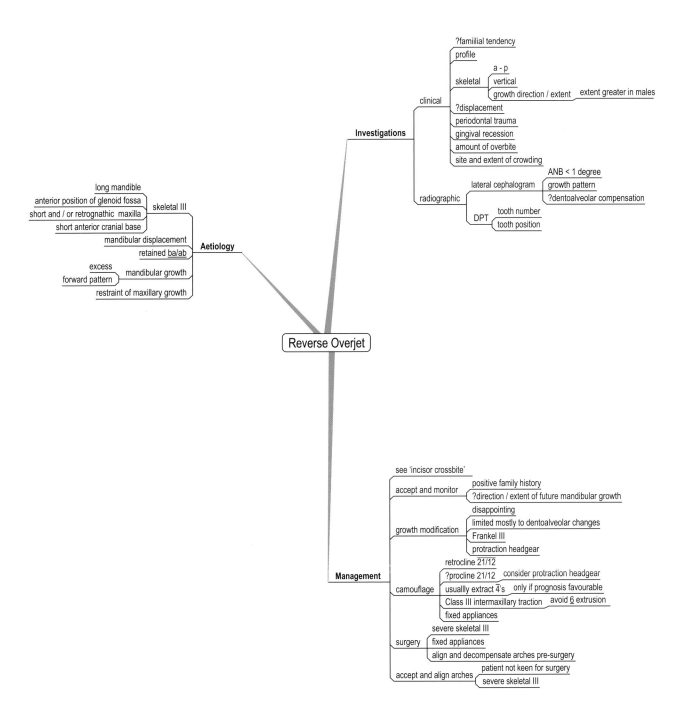

Mind Map 9 Reverse overjet.

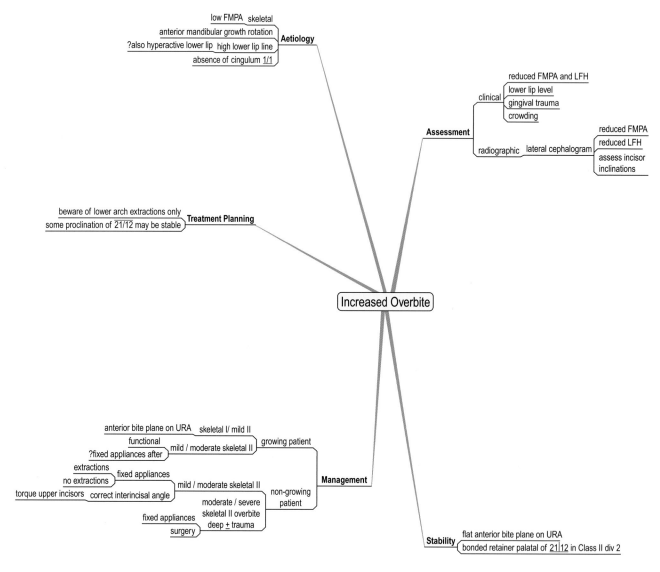

Aetiology
- low FMPA skeletal
- anterior mandibular growth rotation
- ?also hyperactive lower lip high lower lip line
- absence of cingulum 1/1

Assessment
- clinical
  - reduced FMPA and LFH
  - lower lip level
  - gingival trauma
  - crowding
- radiographic lateral cephalogram
  - reduced FMPA
  - reduced LFH
  - assess incisor inclinations

Treatment Planning
- beware of lower arch extractions only
- some proclination of 21/12 may be stable

Management
- growing patient
  - skeletal I/ mild II anterior bite plane on URA
  - mild / moderate skeletal II functional ?fixed appliances after
- non-growing patient
  - mild / moderate skeletal II fixed appliances
    - extractions
    - no extractions
    - torque upper incisors correct interincisal angle
  - moderate / severe skeletal II overbite deep ± trauma
    - fixed appliances
    - surgery

Stability
- flat anterior bite plane on URA
- bonded retainer palatal of 21|12 in Class II div 2

Mind Map 10 Increased overbite.

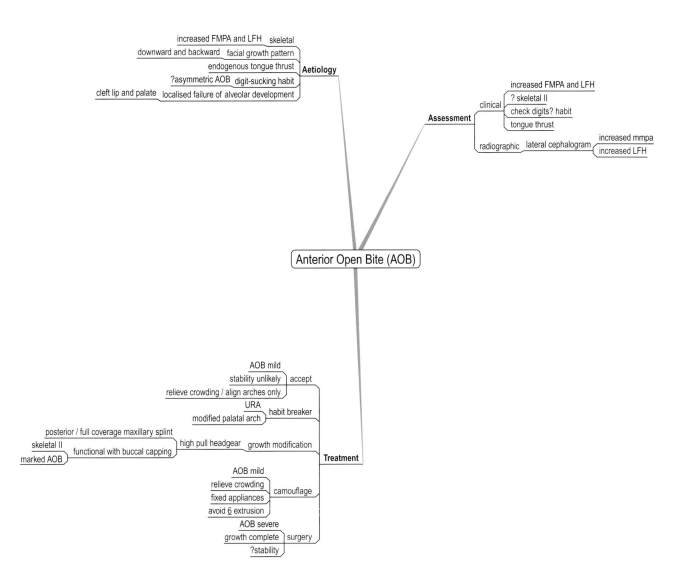

Mind Map 11 Anterior open bite.

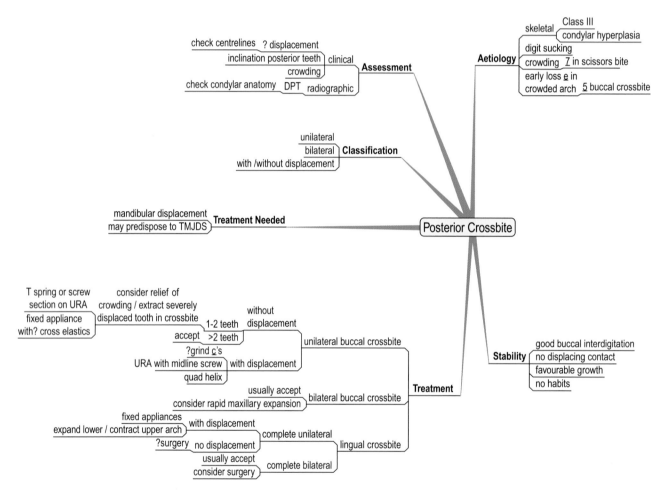

check centrelines ? displacement
inclination posterior teeth | clinical
crowding
check condylar anatomy DPT radiographic **Assessment**

Aetiology
skeletal Class III
condylar hyperplasia
digit sucking
crowding 7 in scissors bite
early loss e in
crowded arch 5 buccal crossbite

unilateral
bilateral **Classification**
with /without displacement

mandibular displacement **Treatment Needed**
may predispose to TMJDS

Posterior Crossbite

T spring or screw   consider relief of
section on URA   crowding / extract severely
fixed appliance   displaced tooth in crossbite
with? cross elastics
                           1-2 teeth without
                           accept >2 teeth displacement
                           ?grind c's
URA with midline screw | with displacement
                           quad helix
                                         unilateral buccal crossbite
                           usually accept
             consider rapid maxillary expansion bilateral buccal crossbite
fixed appliances
expand lower / contract upper arch | with displacement
?surgery no displacement complete unilateral
                           usually accept lingual crossbite
                           consider surgery complete bilateral

Treatment

Stability
good buccal interdigitation
no displacing contact
favourable growth
no habits

Mind Map 12 Posterior crossbite.

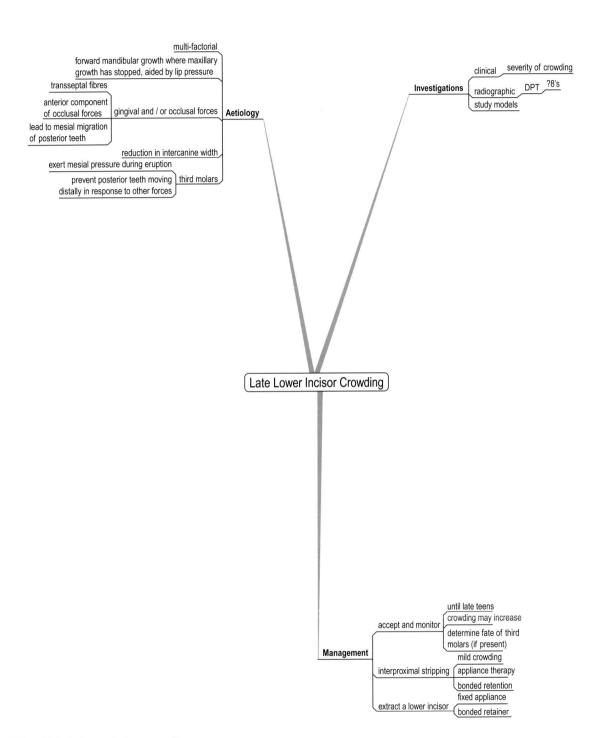

Mind Map 13 Late lower incisor crowding.

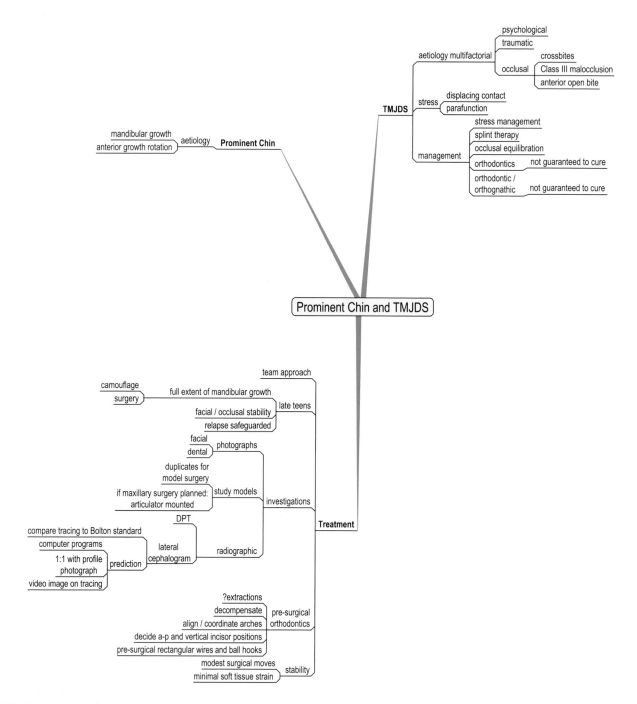

Mind Map 14 Prominent chin and TMJ pain.

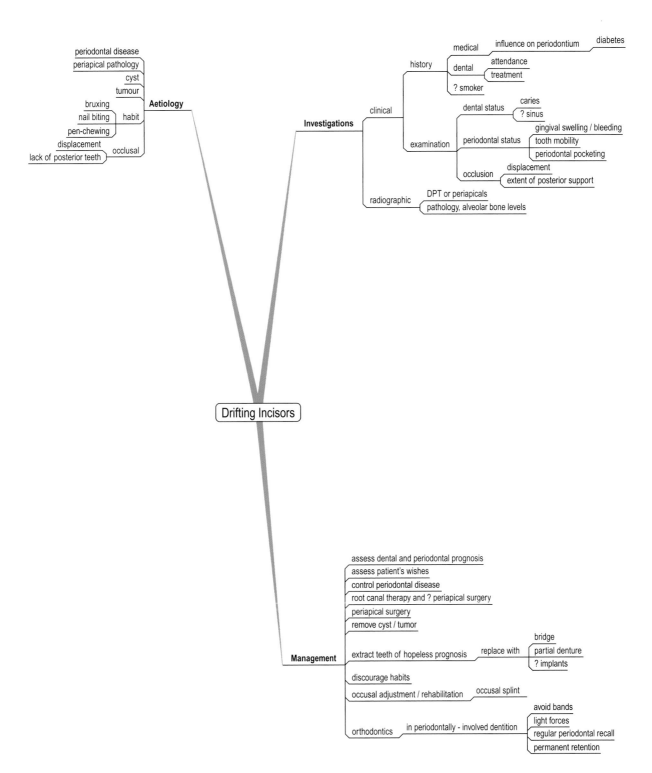

Mind Map 15 Drifting incisors.

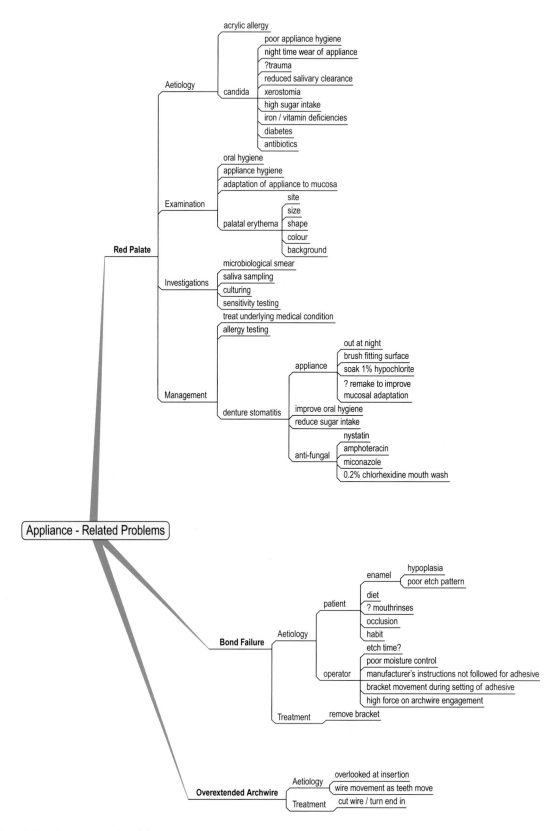

Mind Map 16 Appliance-related problems.

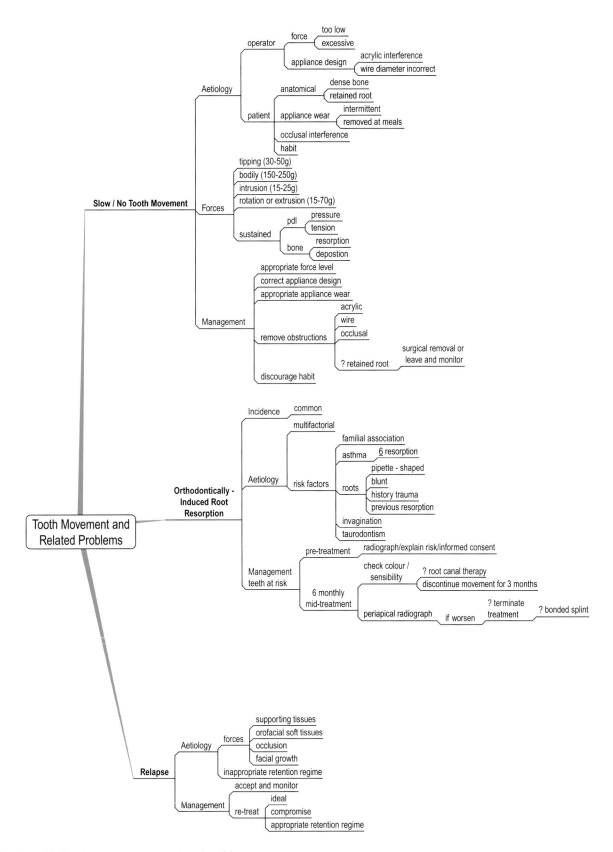

Mind Map 17 Tooth movement and related problems.

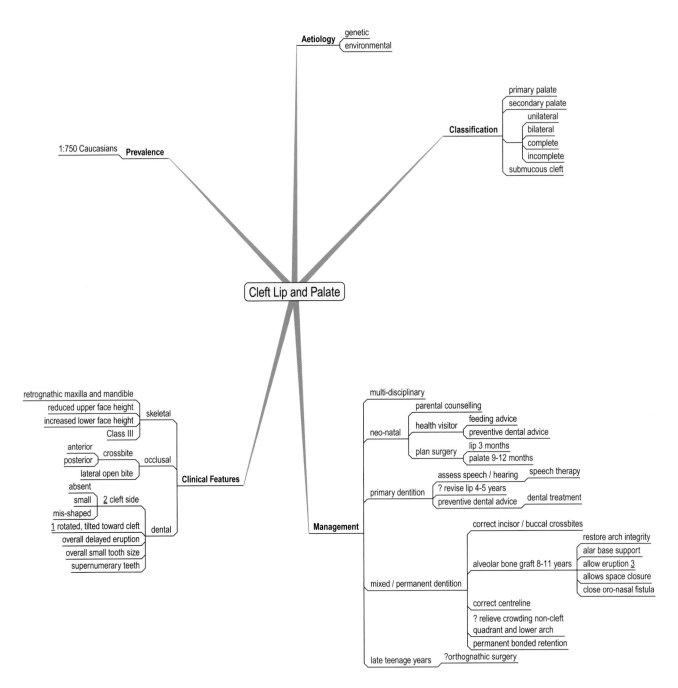

Mind Map 18 Cleft lip and palate.

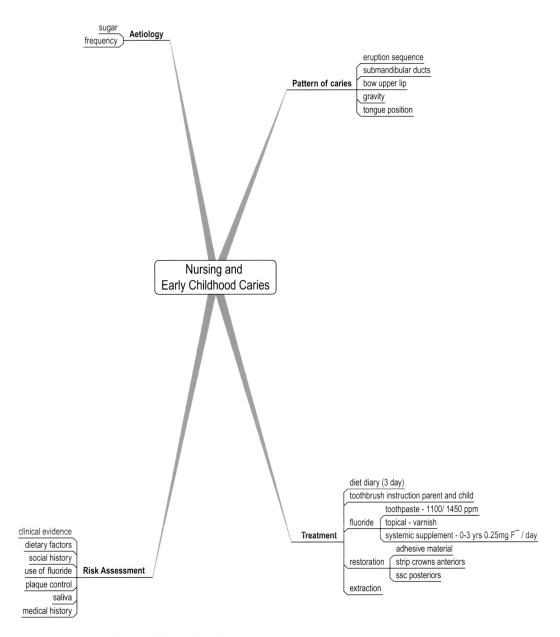

Mind Map 19 Nursing caries and early childhood caries.

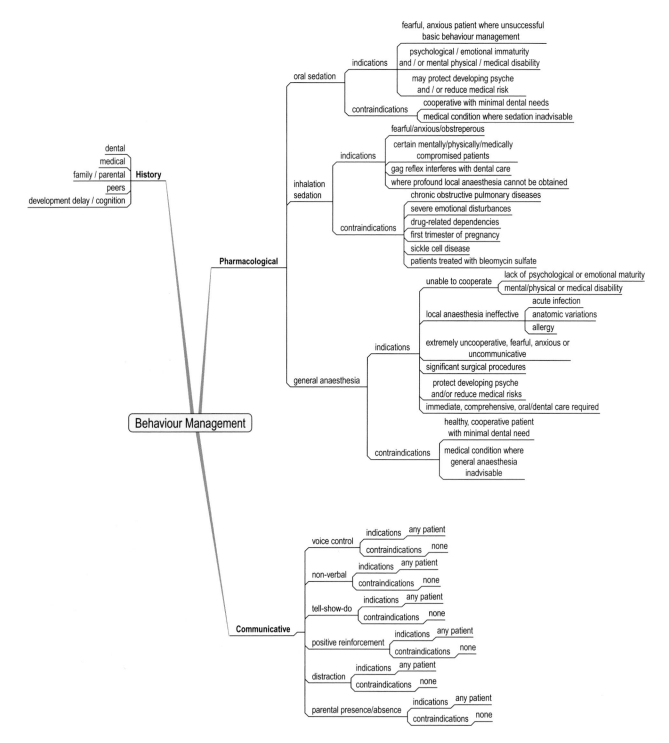

Mind Map 20 Behaviour management

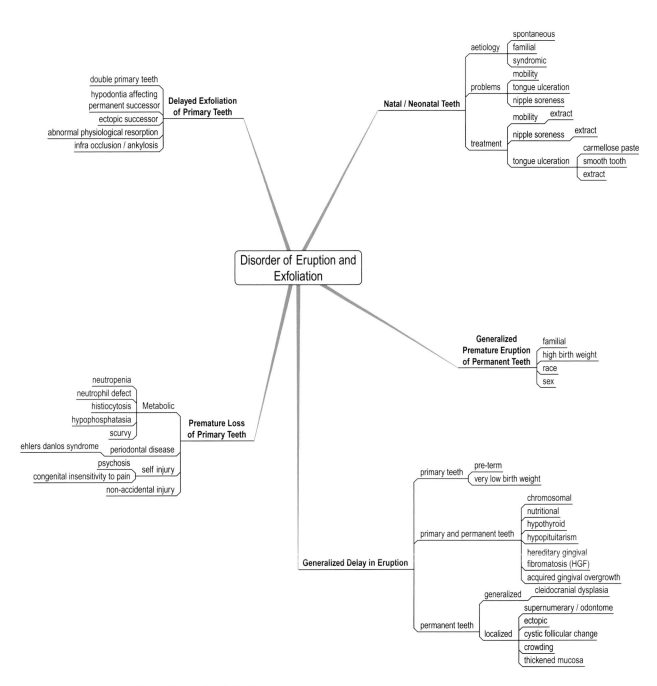

Mind Map 21 Disorders of eruption and exfoliation.

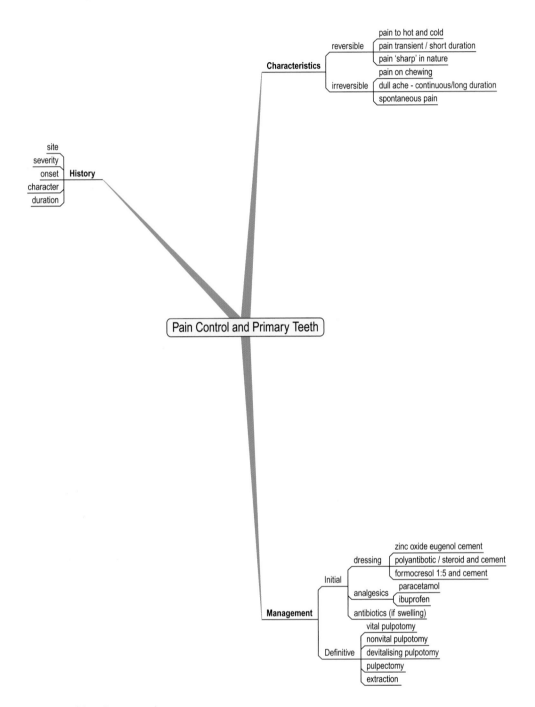

Mind Map 22 Pain control in primary teeth.

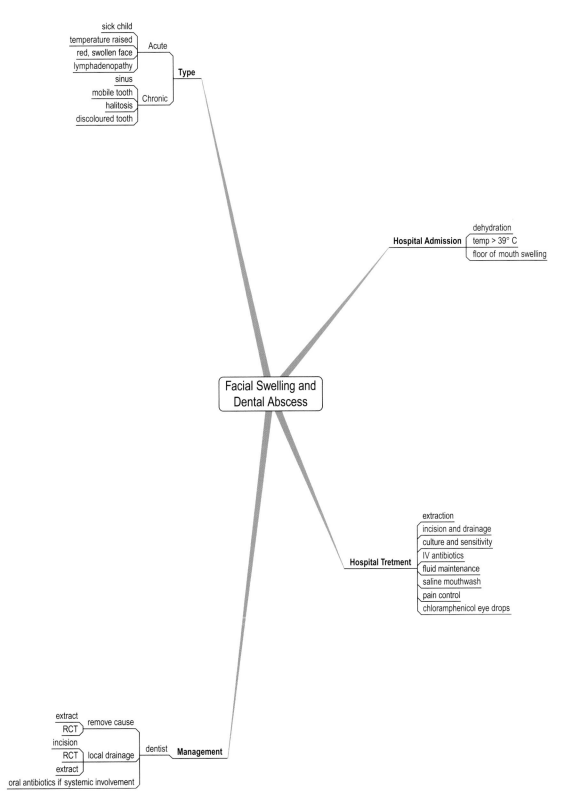

Mind Map 23 Facial swelling and dental abscess.

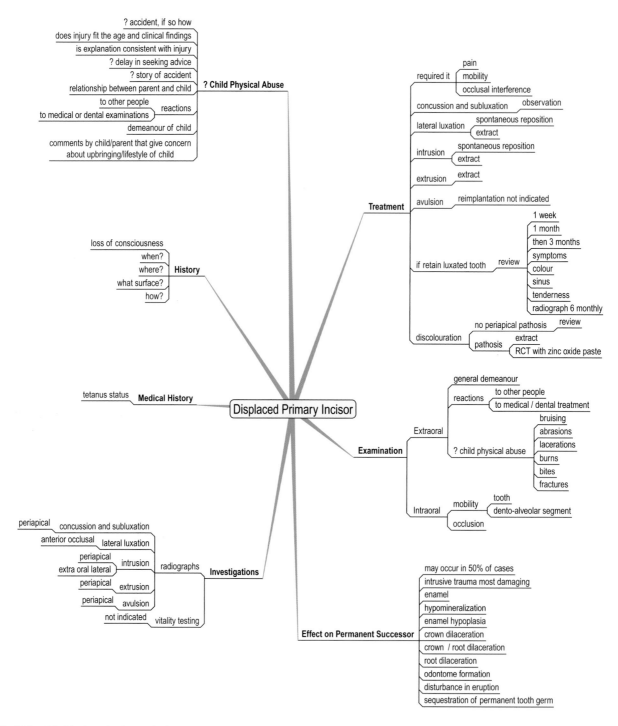

? accident, if so how
does injury fit the age and clinical findings
is explanation consistent with injury
? delay in seeking advice
? story of accident
relationship between parent and child
to other people
to medical or dental examinations — reactions
demeanour of child
comments by child/parent that give concern about upbringing/lifestyle of child

? Child Physical Abuse

required it — pain / mobility / occlusal interference

concussion and subluxation — observation

lateral luxation — spontaneous reposition / extract

intrusion — spontaneous reposition / extract

extrusion — extract

avulsion — reimplantation not indicated

if retain luxated tooth — review — 1 week / 1 month / then 3 months / symptoms / colour / sinus / tenderness / radiograph 6 monthly

discolouration — no periapical pathosis — review / pathosis — extract / RCT with zinc oxide paste

Treatment

loss of consciousness
when?
where?
what surface?
how?

History

tetanus status **Medical History**

Displaced Primary Incisor

Examination

general demeanour
reactions — to other people / to medical / dental treatment
? child physical abuse — bruising / abrasions / lacerations / burns / bites / fractures

Extraoral

Intraoral — mobility — tooth / dento-alveolar segment / occlusion

periapical — concussion and subluxation
anterior occlusal — lateral luxation
periapical / extra oral lateral — intrusion
periapical — extrusion
periapical — avulsion
not indicated — vitality testing

radiographs **Investigations**

Effect on Permanent Successor

may occur in 50% of cases
intrusive trauma most damaging
enamel
hypomineralization
enamel hypoplasia
crown dilaceration
crown / root dilaceration
root dilaceration
odontome formation
disturbance in eruption
sequestration of permanent tooth germ

Mind Map 24 Displaced primary incisor.

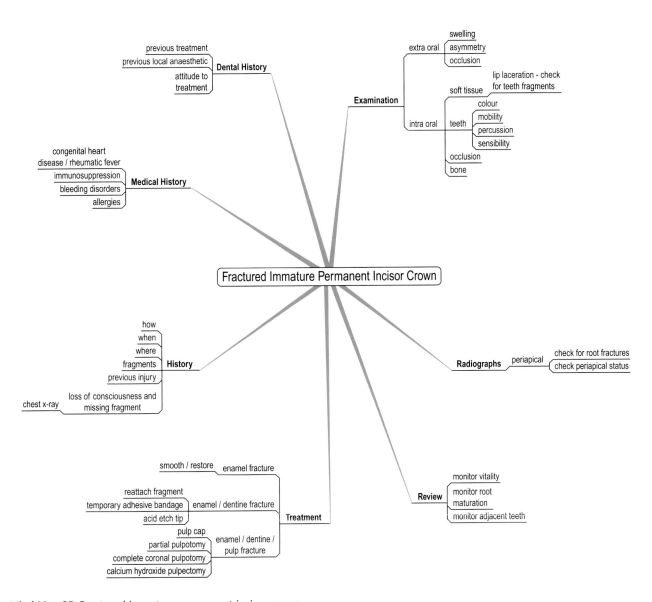

Mind Map 25 Fractured immature permanent incisor crown.

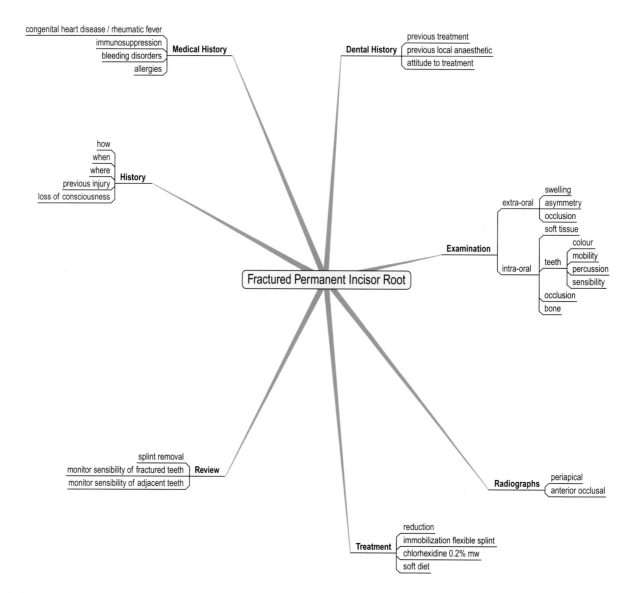

Mind Map 26 Fractured permanent incisor root.

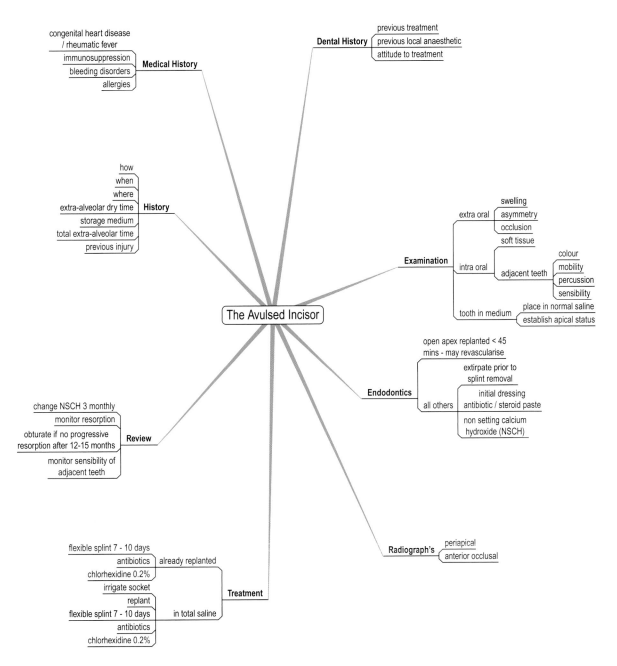

Mind Map 27 The avulsed incisor.

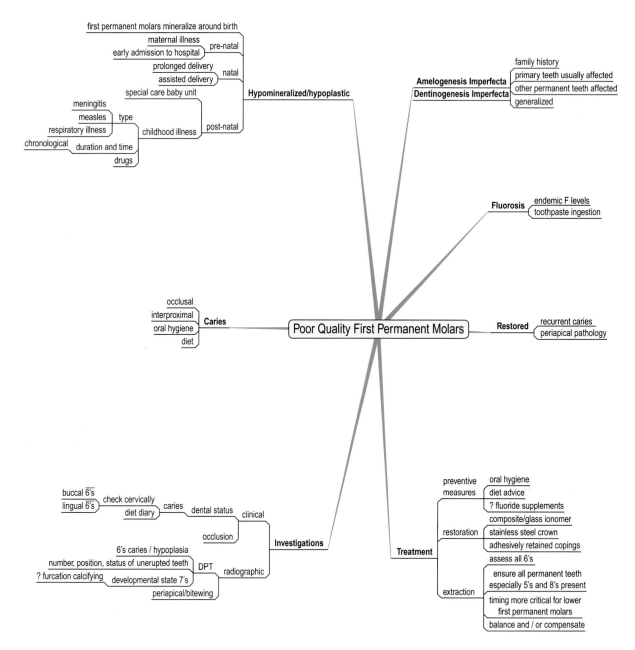

first permanent molars mineralize around birth

maternal illness — pre-natal
early admission to hospital

prolonged delivery — natal
assisted delivery

special care baby unit

meningitis
measles — type
respiratory illness — childhood illness — post-natal
chronological — duration and time
drugs

Hypomineralized/hypoplastic

Amelogenesis Imperfecta
Dentinogenesis Imperfecta
family history
primary teeth usually affected
other permanent teeth affected
generalized

Fluorosis — endemic F levels
toothpaste ingestion

occlusal
interproximal
oral hygiene — **Caries**
diet

Poor Quality First Permanent Molars

Restored — recurrent caries
periapical pathology

buccal 6̄'s
lingual 6̄'s — check cervically — caries
diet diary — dental status — clinical
occlusion

6's caries / hypoplasia
number, position, status of unerupted teeth — DPT — radiographic
? furcation calcifying — developmental state 7's
periapical/bitewing

Investigations

Treatment

preventive measures — oral hygiene
diet advice
? fluoride supplements

restoration — composite/glass ionomer
stainless steel crown
adhesively retained copings

assess all 6's
extraction — ensure all permanent teeth especially 5's and 8's present
timing more critical for lower first permanent molars
balance and / or compensate

Mind Map 28 Poor quality first permanent molars.

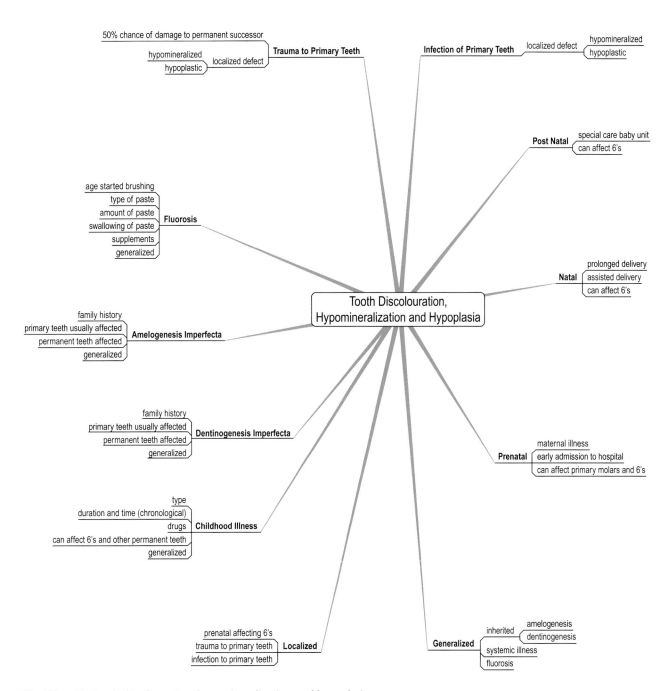

Mind Map 29 Tooth discolouration, hypomineralization and hypoplasia.

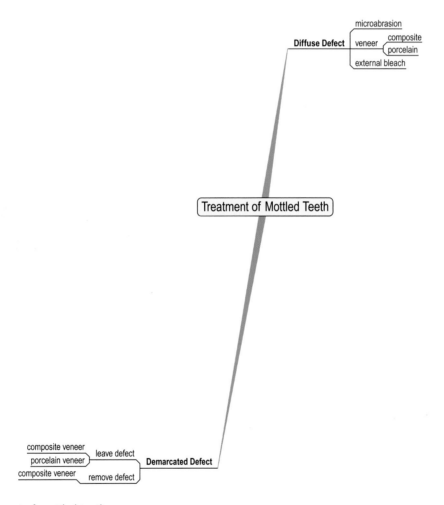

Mind Map 30 Treatment of mottled teeth.

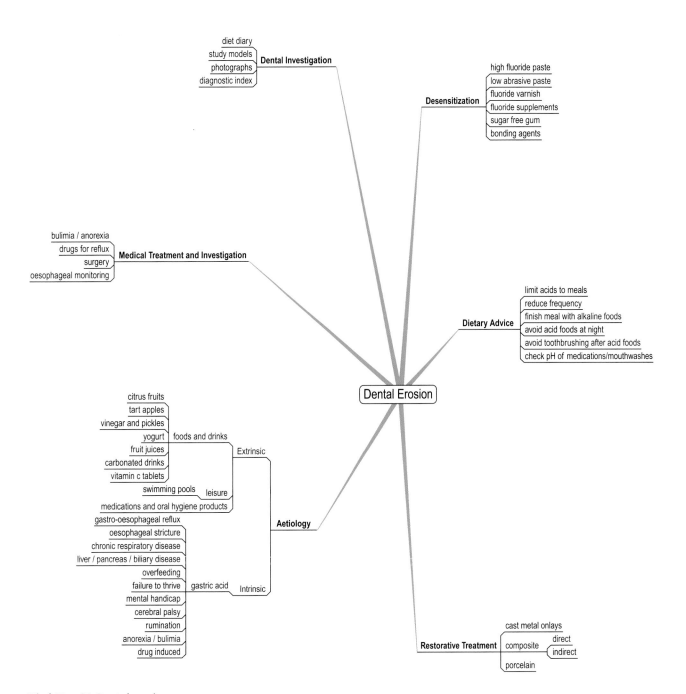

Mind Map 31 Dental erosion.

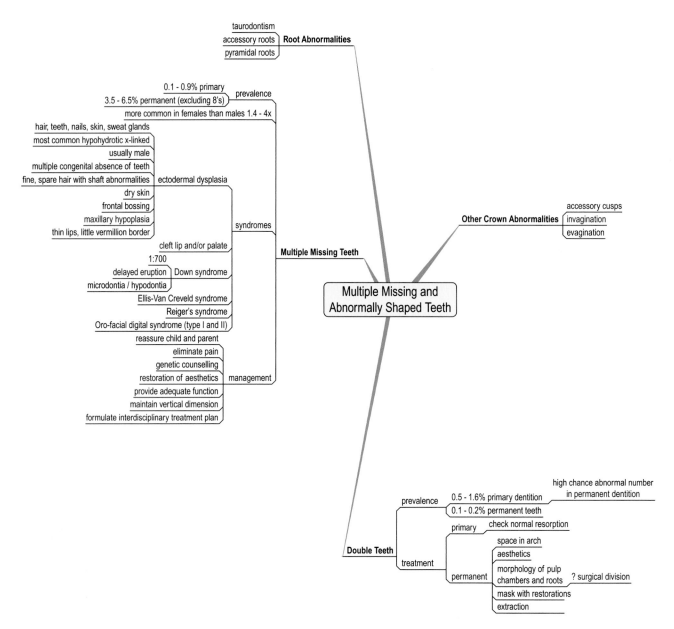

Mind Map 32 Multiple missing and abnormally shaped teeth.

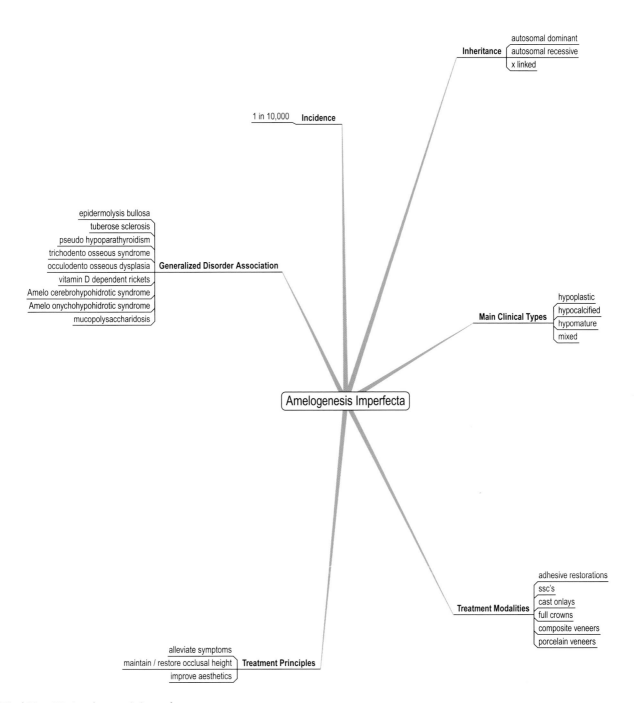

Mind Map 33 Amelogenesis imperfecta.

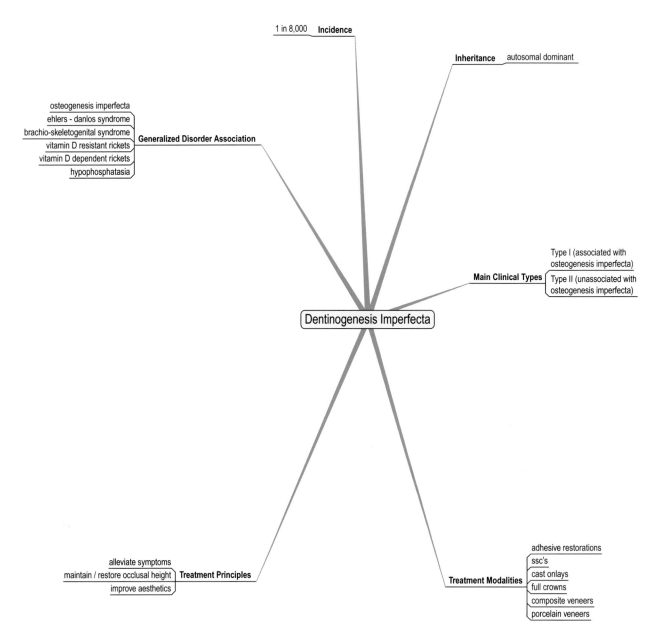

1 in 8,000 **Incidence**

Inheritance autosomal dominant

osteogenesis imperfecta
ehlers - danlos syndrome
brachio-skeletogenital syndrome
vitamin D resistant rickets
vitamin D dependent rickets
hypophosphatasia
Generalized Disorder Association

Main Clinical Types Type I (associated with osteogenesis imperfecta)
Type II (unassociated with osteogenesis imperfecta)

Dentinogenesis Imperfecta

alleviate symptoms
maintain / restore occlusal height
improve aesthetics
Treatment Principles

Treatment Modalities adhesive restorations
ssc's
cast onlays
full crowns
composite veneers
porcelain veneers

Mind Map 34 Dentinogenesis imperfecta.

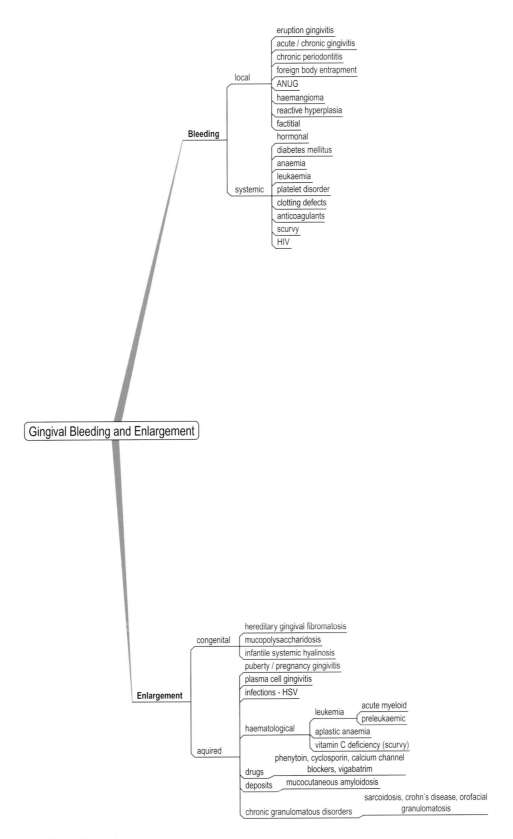

Mind Map 35 Gingival bleeding and enlargement.

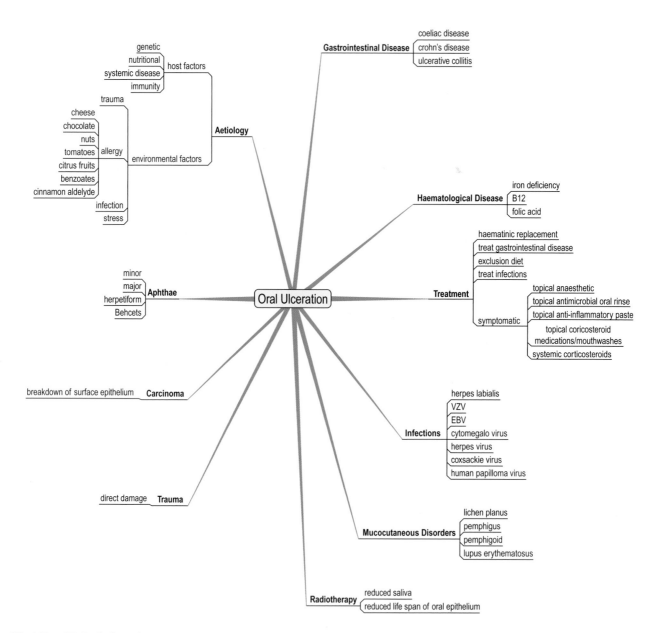

Mind Map 36 Oral ulceration.

A1

The Index of Orthodontic Treatment Need: Dental Health Component

Grade	Characteristics
1 None	Extremely minor malocclusions including displacements <1 mm
2 Little	a. Increased overjet >3.5 mm but ≤6 mm with competent lips
	b. Reverse overjet >0 mm but ≤1 mm
	c. Anterior or posterior crossbite with ≤1 mm discrepancy between retruded contact position and intercuspal position
	d. Displacement of teeth >1 mm but ≤2 mm
	e. Anterior or posterior open bite >1 mm but ≤2 mm
	f. Increased overbite ≥3.5 mm without gingival contact
	g. Prenormal or postnormal occlusions with no other anomalies; includes up to half a unit discrepancy.
3 Moderate	a. Increased overjet >3.5 mm but ≤6 mm with incompetent lips
	b. Reverse overjet >1 mm but ≤3.5 mm
	c. Anterior or posterior crossbites with >1 mm but ≤2 mm discrepancy between retruded contact position and intercuspal position
	d. Displacement of teeth >2 mm but ≤4 mm
	e. Lateral or anterior open bite >2 mm but ≤4 mm
	f. Increased and complete overbite without gingival or palatal trauma
4 Great	a. Increased overjet >6 mm but ≤9 mm
	b. Reverse overjet >3.5 mm with no masticatory or speech difficulties
	c. Anterior or posterior crossbite with >2 mm discrepancy between retruded contact position and intercuspal position
	d. Severe displacements of teeth >4 mm
	e. Extreme lateral or anterior open bites >4 mm
	f. Increased and complete overbite with gingival or palatal trauma
	h. Less extensive hypodontia, requiring prerestorative orthodontics or orthodontic space closure to obviate the need for a prosthesis
	l. Posterior lingual crossbite with no functional occlusal contact in one or both buccal segments
	m. Reverse overjet >1 mm but <3.5 mm, with recorded masticatory and speech difficulties
	t. Partially erupted teeth, tipped and impacted against adjacent teeth
	x. Supplemental teeth
5 Very great	a. Increased overjet >9 mm
	h. Extensive hypodontia with restorative implications (more than one tooth missing in any quadrant) requiring prerestorative orthodontics
	i. Impeded eruption of teeth (with the exception of third molars) owing to crowding, displacement, the presence of supernumerary teeth, retained deciduous teeth and any pathological cause
	m. Reverse overjet >3.5 mm with reported masticatory and speech difficulties
	p. Defects of cleft lip and palate
	s. Submerged deciduous teeth

Reproduced with permission from Heasman P 2003 Master Dentistry Vol 2, Churchill Livingstone, Edinburgh

A2
Lateral cephalometric analysis

Aim and objective of cephalometric analysis

Aim: To assess the anteroposterior and vertical relationships of the upper and lower teeth with supporting alveolar bone to their respective maxillary and mandibular bases and to the cranial base.

Objective: To compare the patient to normal population standards appropriate to their racial group, identifying any differences between the two.

Practice of cephalometric analysis

Ensure that teeth are in occlusion and that the patient is not postured forward.

In a darkened room, by tracing or digitizing, identify the points and planes listed in **Table A2.1** (**Fig. A2.1**); always trace the most prominent image. For structures with two images (e.g. the mandibular border), trace both and take the average for gonion. Calculate angular and linear measurements.

Cephalometric interpretation

For Caucasians, compare individual values with Eastman norms (**Table A2.2**).

Skeletal relationships

A-P. If SNA < or >81° and S–N/Max PL within 8°± 3°, correct ANB as follows: for every °SNA > 81°, subtract 0.5° from ANB value and vice versa.

Vertical. MMPA and Facial % should lend support to each other usually.

Tooth position

- To assess if overjet reduction is possible by tipping movement, do a prognosis tracing (**Fig. A2.2**), or for every 1 mm of overjet reduction subtract 2.5° from $\underline{1}$ inclination. If the final inclination is not <95° to maxillary plane, tipping is acceptable.
- Check $\overline{1}$ angulation to mandibular plane in conjunction with ANB and MMPA. There is an inverse relationship between $\overline{1}$ angulation and MMPA.
- Interincisal angle: as this increases, overbite deepens.
- $\overline{1}$ to APo: this is an aesthetic reference line but it is unwise to use for treatment planning purposes.

Soft tissue analysis

- *Holdaway line*: lower lip should be ± 1 mm to this line.
- *Ricketts' E-line*: lower lip should be 0 mm (±2 mm) in front of this with the upper lip slightly behind (**Fig. A2.3**).

Table A2.1 Definition of commonly used cephalometric points and planes

	Definition
Points	
S	sella: midpoint of sella turcica
N	nasion: most anterior point of the frontonasal suture (may use the deepest point at the junction of the frontal and nasal bones instead)
P	porion: uppermost, outermost point on the bony external auditory meatus (upper border of the condylar head is at the same level, which helps location)
O	orbitale: most inferior anterior point on the margin of the orbit (use average of the left and right orbital shadows)
ANS	tip of the anterior nasal spine
PNS	tip of the posterior nasal spine (pterygomaxillary fissure is directly above, which helps location)
A	A point: most posterior point of the concavity on the anterior surface of the premaxilla in the midline below ANS
B	B point: most posterior point of the concavity on the anterior surface of the mandible in the midline above pogonion
Pog	pogonion: most anterior point on the bony chin
Me	menton: lowermost point on the mandibular symphysis in the midline
Go	gonion: most posterio-inferior point at the angle of the mandible (bisect the angle between tangent to the posterior ramus and inferior body of the mandible to locate)
Planes S–N line	line drawn through S and N
Frankfort plane	line connecting porion and orbitale
Maxillary plane	line joining PNS and ANS
Mandibular plane	line joining Go to Me
Functional occlusal plane	line drawn between the cusp tips of the first permanent molars and premolars/primary molars

Reproduced with permission from Heasman P 2003 Master Dentistry Vol 2, Churchill Livingstone, Edinburgh

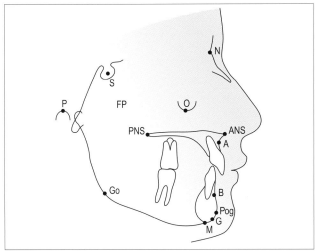

Fig. A2.1 Standard cephalometric points. Adapted from: Heasman 2003, Master Dentistry Vol 2. Restorative dentistry, paediatric dentistry and orthodontics. Churchill Livingstone, Edinburgh.

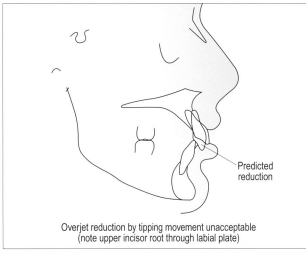

Overjet reduction by tipping movement unacceptable
(note upper incisor root through labial plate)

Fig. A2.2 Prognosis tracing.

Table A2.2 Normal Eastman cephalometric values for Caucasians

Parameter	Value (± SD)
SNA	81 ± 3°
SNB	78 ± 3°
ANB	3 ± 2°
S–N/Max	8 ± 3°
$\bar{1}$ to Maxillary Pl	109 ± 6°
$\bar{1}$ to Mandibular Pl	93 ± 6°
Interincisal angle	135 ± 10°
MMPA	27 ± 4°
Facial proportion	55 ± 2%

Reproduced with permission from Heasman P 2003 Master Dentistry Vol 2, Churchill Livingstone, Edinburgh

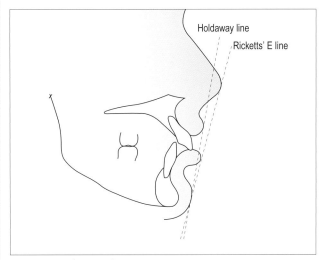

Fig. A2.3 Soft tissue lines.

Index